Rural Surgery

Editor

TYLER G. HUGHES

SURGICAL CLINICS OF NORTH AMERICA

www.surgical.theclinics.com

Consulting Editor
RONALD F. MARTIN

October 2020 • Volume 100 • Number 5

ELSEVIER

1600 John F. Kennedy Boulevard • Suite 1800 • Philadelphia, Pennsylvania, 19103-2899

http://www.surgical.theclinics.com

SURGICAL CLINICS OF NORTH AMERICA Volume 100, Number 5
October 2020 ISSN 0039-6109, ISBN-13: 978-0-323-79492-3

Editor: John Vassallo, j.vassallo@elsevier.com
Developmental Editor: Nicole Congleton

Surgical Clinics of North America (ISSN 0039-6109) is published bimonthly by Elsevier Inc., 360 Park Avenue South, New York, NY 10010-1710. Months of publication are February, April, June, August, October, and December. Business and Editorial Offices: 1600 John F. Kennedy Blvd., Suite 1800, Philadelphia, PA 19103-2899. Periodicals postage paid at New York, NY and additional mailing offices. Subscription prices are $430.00 per year for US individuals, $891.00 per year for US institutions, $100.00 per year for US & Canadian students and residents, $507.00 per year for Canadian individuals, $1130.00 per year for Canadian institutions, $536.00 for international individuals, $1130.00 per year for international institutions and $250.00 per year for foreign students/residents. To receive student/resident rate, orders must be accompanied by name of affiliated institution, date of term, and the *signature* of program/residency coordinator on institution letterhead. Orders will be billed at individual rate until proof of status is received. Foreign air speed delivery is included in all *Clinics* subscription prices. All prices are subject to change without notice. POSTMASTER: Send address changes to *Surgical Clinics*, Elsevier Health Sciences Division, Subscription Customer Service, 3251 Riverport Lane, Maryland Heights, MO 63043. **Customer Service (orders, claims, online, change of address): Telephone: 1-800-654-2452 (U.S. and Canada); 314-447-8871 (outside U.S. and Canada). Fax: 314-447-8029. E-mail: journalscustomerservice-usa@elsevier.com (for print support); journalsonlinesupport-usa@elsevier.com (for online support)**.

Reprints. For copies of 100 or more, of articles in this publication, please contact the Commercial Reprints Department, Elsevier Inc., 360 Park Avenue South, New York, New York 10010-1710. Tel. 212-633-3874, Fax: 212-633-3820, E-mail: reprints@elsevier.com.

The Surgical Clinics of North America is also published in Spanish by McGraw-Hill Interamericana Editores S.A., P.O. Box 5-237 06500 Mexico D.F. Mexico; and in Portuguese by Interlivros Edicoes Ltda., Rua Comandante Coelho 1085, CEP 21250, Rio de Janeiro, Brazil; and in Greek by Paschalidis Medical Publications, Athens Greece.

The Surgical Clinics of North America is covered in *MEDLINE/PubMed (Index Medicus), EMBASE/Excerpta Medica, Current Contents/Clinical Medicine, Current Contents/Life Sciences, Science Citation Index*, and *ISI/BIOMED*.

Contributors

CONSULTING EDITOR

RONALD F. MARTIN, MD, FACS
Colonel (Retired), United States Army Reserve, Executive Vice President, Kalispell, Regional Healthcare, Chief Physician Executive, Kalispell Regional Medical Group, Division of HPB Surgery and Surgical Oncology, Kalispell, Montana

EDITOR

TYLER G. HUGHES, MD, FACS
Clinical Professor of Surgery, Director of Medical Education, University of Kansas School of Medicine, Salina Campus, Salina, Kansas

AUTHORS

MARY OLINE AALAND, MD, FACS
Department of Surgery, University of North Dakota, Grand Forks, North Dakota

JOANNA VEAZEY BROOKS, MBE, PhD
Assistant Professor, Department of Population Health, University of Kansas School of Medicine, Kansas City, Kansas

KAYLA J. BURCHILL, MD, FACS
Clinical Assistant Professor, Assistant Director of Surgical Education, Department of Surgery, University of North Dakota School of Medicine and Health Sciences, Grand Forks, North Dakota

JULIE CONYERS, MD, MBA, FACS
Department of Surgery, PeaceHealth Ketchikan, Ketchikan, Alaska

ADRIAN DIAZ, MD, MPH
Division of Surgical Oncology, The Ohio State University Wexner Medical Center and James Comprehensive Cancer Center, Columbus, Ohio; National Clinician Scholars Program at the Institute for Healthcare Policy and Innovation, Center for Healthcare Outcomes and Policy, University of Michigan, Ann Arbor, Michigan

AMY L. HALVERSON, MD, MHPE, FACS, FASCRS
Professor of Surgery, Northwestern University Feinberg School of Medicine, Chicago, Illinois

DOROTHY HUGHES, MHSA, PhD
Assistant Professor, Departments of Population Health and Surgery, University of Kansas School of Medicine, Kansas City, Kansas

MELISSA K. JOHNSON, MD, FACS
Associate Professor and Associate Program Director, Department of Surgery, USD Sanford School of Medicine, Royal C. Johnson Veterans Memorial Hospital, Sioux Falls, South Dakota

STEFAN W. JOHNSON, MD, FACS
Clinical Assistant Professor, Program Director, Department of Surgery, University of North Dakota School of Medicine and Health Sciences, Grand Forks, North Dakota

MEGAN NELSON, MD, FACS
Chair, Division of Community General Surgery, Consultant, Department of Trauma, Critical Care and General Surgery, Assistant Program Director, General Surgery Residency Program, Mayo Clinic, Rochester, Minnesota

TIMOTHY M. PAWLIK, MD, MPH, MTS, PhD, FACS, FRACS (Hon)
Center for Healthcare Outcomes and Policy, University of Michigan, Ann Arbor, Michigan; Professor and Chair, Department of Surgery, The Urban Meyer III and Shelley Meyer Chair for Cancer Research, Professor of Surgery, Oncology, Health Services Management and Policy, The Ohio State University, Wexner Medical Center, Columbus, Ohio

RIANN ROBBINS, MD
Surgical Resident, Department of Surgery, University of Utah, Salt Lake City, Utah

MICHAEL ROSKOS, MD, FACS
Consultant, Department of General Surgery, Mayo Clinic La Crosse Fransican Healthcare, La Crosse, Wisconsin; Assistant Program Director, Track General Surgery Residency Program, Mayo Clinic Integrated Community and Rural Surgery, Assistant Professor, Mayo Clinic, Rochester, Minnesota

JARRON M. SAINT ONGE, PhD
Department of Sociology, University of Kansas, Lawrence, Kansas; Department of Population Health, University of Kansas Medical Center, Kansas City, Kansas

MICHAEL DUKE SARAP, MD, FACS
Chair, SE Med Department of Surgery, Cambridge, Ohio; Chair, American College of Surgeons, Advisory Council for Rural Surgery, Co-Chair, Commission on Cancer Program in Ohio, Clinical Professor, Department of Surgery, Wright State University Boonshoft School of Medicine, Dayton, Ohio; Clinical Instructor, Lake Erie College of Medicine, Erie, Pennsylvania; Clinical Instructor, Physicians Assistant Program, Marietta College, Chair, Tina Kiser Cancer Concern Coalition

SARAH SMITH, MA
Department of Sociology, University of Kansas, Lawrence, Kansas

ROBERT P. STICCA, MD, FACS
Professor and Chairman, Department of Surgery, University of North Dakota School of Medicine and Health Sciences, Grand Forks, North Dakota

THAVAM C. THAMBI-PILLAI, MD, MBA, FACS
Professor and Program Director, Department of Surgery, USD Sanford School of Medicine, Sanford Medical Center, Sioux Falls, South Dakota

GARY L. TIMMERMAN, MD, FACS
Professor and Chair, Department of Surgery, USD Sanford School of Medicine, Sanford Medical Center, Sioux Falls, South Dakota

JOHN PATRICK WALKER, MD, FACS
Professor, James C. Thompson Distinguished Chair, Department of Surgery, The University of Texas Medical Branch, Galveston, Texas

JOHN A. WEIGELT, DVM, MD, MMA, FACS
Professor, Department of Surgery, USD Sanford School of Medicine, Sioux Falls, South Dakota

RANDALL ZUCKERMAN, MD, FACS
Chairman, Department of Surgery, Kalispell Regional Medical Center, Kalispell Regional Healthcare, Kailispell, Montana

Contents

Foreword: The Challenges within Rural Surgery xiii

Ronald F. Martin

Preface: Rural Surgery: Then, Now, and Beyond xvii

Tyler G. Hughes

Demographics in Rural Populations 823

Jarron M. Saint Onge and Sarah Smith

This article reviews key population trends affecting rural American health. The article explains the role of demography in defining and studying rural health using example data from the 2014 to 2018 American Community Survey. Specific trends, including depopulation, aging, racial/ethnic diversification, socioeconomic status, and health characteristics found in rural areas, are highlighted. Insights are offered into how population trends, changing age and sex structures, and socioeconomic distributions have implications for rural health care practitioners and surgeons. Several areas and opportunities to address current and future rural health needs are identified.

Rural Surgery and Status of the Rural Workplace: Hospital Survival and Economics 835

Adrian Diaz and Timothy M. Pawlik

Nearly 60 million people live in a rural area across the United States. Since 2005, 162 rural hospitals have closed, and the rate of rural hospital closures seems to be accelerating. Major drivers of rural hospital closures are poor financial health, aging facilities, and low occupancy rates. Rural hospitals are particularly vulnerable to policy and market changes, and even small changes can have a disproportionate effect on rural hospital financial viability. Surgery can be safely performed in rural hospitals; however, hospital closures may be putting the rural population at increased risk of morbidity and mortality from surgical disease.

Initial and Ongoing Training of the Rural Surgeon 849

Gary L. Timmerman, Thavam C. Thambi-Pillai, Melissa K. Johnson, and John A. Weigelt

Over the last 2 decades, rural locations have realized a steady decrease in surgical access and direct care. Owing to societal expectations for equal general and subspecialty surgical care in urban or rural areas, the ability to attract, train, and hold onto the rural surgeon has come into question. Our current general surgery training curriculum has been reevaluated as to its relevance for rural surgery and several alternatives to the traditional surgical training model have been proposed. The authors discuss and evaluate current and proposed methods for surgical training curriculums and methods for rural surgeon retention through continuing education models.

within the context of the rural community and outcomes analyzed with relevant risk adjustment for patient factors.

Advanced Technology and the Rural Surgeon 909

Robert P. Sticca, Kayla J. Burchill, and Stefan W. Johnson

Advanced technology has resulted in major changes in surgery and medicine over the past three decades. There are many barriers to the adoption of advanced technologies, which can be more prevalent in rural hospitals and surgical practices. Despite barriers to implementation of new technologies in rural communities, many rural hospitals have endorsed and invested in these technologies for the benefit of the hospital and community. The rural surgeon is often the driving force in evaluating and deciding on new technologies for their surgical program. This article discusses advantages, challenges, and limitations in the use of advanced technologies in rural locations.

Dealing with the Sick Rural Surgery Patient in Need of Transfer 921

Julie Conyers

Care for rural and urban surgical patients is increasingly more complex due to advancing knowledge and technology. Interhospital transfers occur in approximately 10% of index encounters at rural hospitals secondary to mismatch of patient needs and local resources. Due to the recent expansion of air transport to rural areas, distance and geography are less of a barrier. The interhospital transfer process is understudied and far from standardized. Interhospital transfer status is associated with increase in mortality, complications, length of stay, and costs. The cost, price to patients, and safety of air ambulance transports cannot be ignored.

Regionalization of General Surgery Within the Mayo Clinic Health System and the Mayo Clinic 937

Michael Roskos and Megan Nelson

Regionalization of surgery is an important component of surgical outcomes. This has been based on numerous studies validating the relationship of surgical volume to surgical outcomes. The Mayo Clinic is actively engaged in regionalization of surgery within its health system. It has embraced a nonvolume outcome approach focusing on outcomes using electronic medical record data mining and National Surgical Quality Improvement Program. Implementing surgical regionalization is supported but ineffectively implemented. In addition, the implementation process has been poorly described in the literature. The Mayo clinic has actively implemented regionalization within its health system, which includes supporting the health system.

Using Qualitative Research to Study the Profession of Rural Surgery 949

Dorothy Hughes and Joanna Veazey Brooks

This is a systematic review of original research articles that use qualitative methods to investigate rural surgery over the last decade (2010–2019). This review found that interviews and focus groups were common, most

often engaging with patients and health care professionals. Thematic analysis and grounded theory were data analysis methods most frequently used among these qualitative rural surgery studies. Studies in this review often pertained to obstetrics or the provision of other other surgical services. Areas for future qualitative research on rural surgery are surgical teamwork, scope of practice, workforce shortages, and issues related to the aging rural patient.

SURGICAL CLINICS OF NORTH AMERICA

FORTHCOMING ISSUES

December 2020
Endoscopic Surgery
John H. Rodriguez and Jeffrey L. Ponsky, *Editors*

February 2021
Patient Safety
Feibi Zheng, *Editor*

April 2021
Emerging Bariatric Surgical Procedures
Shanu N. Kothari, *Editor*

RECENT ISSUES

August 2020
Wound Management
Michael D. Caldwell and Michael J. Harl, *Editors*

June 2020
Surgical Oncology for the General Surgeon
Randall Zuckerman and Neal Wilkinson, *Editors*

April 2020
Robotic Surgery
Julio A. Teixeira, *Editor*

Foreword
The Challenges within Rural Surgery

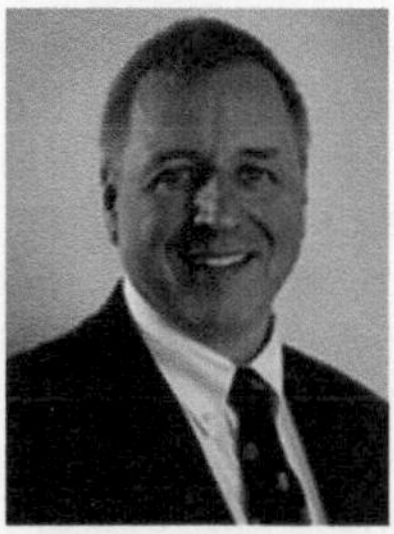

Ronald F. Martin, MD, FACS
Consulting Editor

Many of you as you went through training in medical school, residency, or elsewhere may have heard the statement that people are divided into 2 groups when it comes to problem diagnosing: lumpers and splitters. I think a majority of surgeons tend more toward the "lumper" category as we frequently have to make decisions with incomplete data. As those of you who have read the forewords in the *Surgical Clinics* may have noticed, I tend to lump not just diagnoses of clinical processes but somewhat extend the problems we face as physicians and members of the health care industry to society at large. This foreword will be no exception to that. The topic we need to examine as we prepare to consider the issues facing rural surgery is that of *reserve* or perhaps the lack thereof.

As of the writing of this issue, we are finding our way through the middle of the pandemic's transition from first wave to whatever we will agree to call the period when reopening led to and/or coincided with a resurgence of viral cases. Multiple analyses are being posited by the lay press about the similarities of disease spread of COVID-19 and our ability in the United States to respond to the disease comparing the period of mid-April 2020 with the period of early to mid-July 2020. Some of those comparisons are fairer than others. While the case number rises are reminiscent, the lethality is a bit different as are the hospitalizations, depending on where you look geographically. There may be good reasons for this difference. Perhaps we are better capable of detecting, isolating, and treating patients who are sick now than we were a few months ago. Perhaps testing is more available than it was, even if not as available as we would like. Perhaps younger people have led the charge of being the infected group as the weather warmed. Even if all those factors are at play, the factor that is likely more impactful in the difference between prevalence and lethality is reserve.

It was not that long ago, a few decades, that hospitals had physical stockpiles of supplies, had ample amounts of days-in-cash (that were intended to be used for

Surg Clin N Am 100 (2020) xiii–xvi
https://doi.org/10.1016/j.suc.2020.07.005

emergency, not to prop up bond ratings), had adequate personnel in reserve to supplement staffing, and had available beds for surge capacity. These systems were less efficient than the ones we have now. With hospitals now functioning much more like other non–health care corporations, the ever-increasing demand for short-term financial performance and maximizing profit (spelled "margin" if you work for a 501c3 but treated pretty much just the same as for-profit entities treat profit), the reserves of these systems have been eroded.

Since the widespread adoption of the Internet that provided us with Amazon.com and other companies who sell via the Internet, along with their global supply chains, the idea of keeping inventory on hand when it can be ordered "just-in-time" has markedly vanished. Keeping on "expensive" full-time staff when one could use short-term temporary staffing to bolster periodic needs has been considered a cost too high. An empty hospital bed might be just as easily looked at as a poor productivity metric rather than as a strategic reserve. In short, many hospitals and health care organizations have stripped down their systems of "dead weight" in order to improve financial performance.

Hospital-based platforms and health care systems are not alone in this regard. The overwhelming majority of people in the United States act in a similar fashion. I have heard estimates that more than 95% of people in the United States would have to sell something to handle a short-term financial burden—like getting ill, for example. Many people have little to no financial reserve at home in case their job suddenly goes away.

Companies similarly rely on cheaper labor and products from the global supply chain assuming these chains will be adequately reliable—and if not, one can buy from another country who will provide cheap labor. These same companies who rely on just-in-time global supply chains frequently live and die financially based on quarterly reports. If they are publicly traded, they are forever hostage to algorithmic machine trading on the various exchanges, which magnify the effect of disruptive events in their business models.

All in all, as grim as the above may sound, it has actually worked pretty well for the past several years to few decades. It is a remarkable and remarkably connected system that allows many to benefit from the ability to transmit information and money instantly. As a result, companies can use this network to meet our collective needs. It should always work like a charm unless one thing happens—the whole system breaks at once.

Pandemics are fundamentally different from most catastrophic events in one major way. In most disasters, we try to colocate people and resources to improve our ability to cope. We increase personal contact and facilitate the movement of needed supplies. In pandemics, we try to dislocate and diffuse people as much as we can in order to prevent transmission of disease. We also disrupt travel and transport of goods. Diffusion and lack of contact by their very nature generate less efficient systems. Everyone needs to shelter in place with their stockpile to weather the problem. We can't rely on one another for shared efficiencies. Panic buying begins along with hoarding on occasion. Disputes as to what services are essential and disruptions to workforce—either from disease or from competing burdens for family care—further decrease overall system efficiency.

All of these things mentioned above happened to hospital systems just as they did to other industries and to households, though, in addition, hospitals were expected to make ready for an unprecedented and unpredictable need for medical care secondary to a single disease process. In other words, hospitals had to spend a lot of money to prepare for a disease that may or not come their way in a hypercompetitive sellers' market for supplies. All while halting the activity that brought in revenue in the first place. This last consideration is what brings us back to the concept of rural hospitals. Rural hospitals struggle to maintain resource capability for their constituent populations all the time. The main pressure relief valve is to transfer a patient who needs greater resources to a facility with greater capability. When those higher-echelon levels of care either lose capability (beds or staffing) or lose their ability to purchase supplies, the whole system begins to crumble. When every facility has to fend for itself, the rural hospitals are frequently the least financially capable of handling the burden—even if help from other agencies is imminent.

Over the years, larger hospital organizations, for various reasons, did not maintain their reserves of people, beds, or supplies. In my opinion, perhaps many of them felt that it was the responsibility of others to be prepared for such a calamity. In the case of one or a few hospitals suddenly being taxed by demand, the option to transfer patients or borrow supplies always seemed to be there. Or perhaps, it was felt that the government should be able to provide the required missing elements at low cost or no cost in unexpected situations. I can't say I disagree with the concepts. One description of a government is that it is an insurance company with an army. I'll grant that description is woefully incomplete, but there is some truth to it. The federal government, in the United States anyway, represents the last line of the collective "we the people." If the collective resources of all of us can't solve a problem, then there is truly big trouble.

A funny thing happened on the way to the National Strategic Stockpiles. We found out upon arrival that our strategic reserves were small fractions of what we believed them to be. We then turned to manufacturing and found out that our ability to "just-in-time" order was profoundly constrained, and our ability to "just-in-time" produce goods was crippled as well. The rest of the world found themselves in similar positions. In short, we had no reserve.

For rural hospitals to survive, they either need to achieve enough "critical mass" of their own to weather storms such as these or they need to be integrated into larger systems with such capacities. Both strategies are challenging when you compare the current structures for critical access hospitals and the differing structures for prospective payment system hospitals. It gets worse when you take into account for-profit and not-for-profit entities. Even if we were to amalgamate these rural care sites with larger organizations in some way, that would not assure that we would be better positioned in the future for unexpected demand in the future. After all, neither the large systems nor the state or federal governments were remotely prepared for this latest challenge. To be fair, nobody was prepared.

We could be prepared. I am not sure that we will, but we could be. We could understand the challenges to deliver health care to austere or low-population-density environments. We could understand how to best develop and maintain strategic supplies of equipment, medicines, and personnel. We could develop state and regional agreements with the federal government for sharing the burdens and providing for rapid distribution of scarce supplies. We could find a way to support higher levels of strategic preparedness for the larger or higher-capability health care centers to stop them from going broke if they tried to do so. We could revisit the nature of medicine as a business in the United States to assure that we have a system that is capable of delivering on its many promises. We could.

As with so many things, if you want to make progress, you have to understand the challenge. In this issue of the *Surgical Clinics*, Dr Tyler Hughes and his colleagues have prepared an excellent collection of reviews that will help any reader to better understand the capabilities and the challenges that rural hospitals have. I am deeply indebted to Dr Hughes for his efforts. He is valued colleague and a cherished friend of mine as well as of the entire surgical community.

At the *Surgical Clinics*, we have maintained a philosophy that we wish to deliver content in context. We wish to have breadth and depth in our writings and provide our readership with a product that will not just answer some immediate question but also provide the material to delve deeper into the mastery of the topic. We wish to provide the ability for people to find answers—or at least direction—to questions they haven't thought to ask yet. I encourage the reader to consume these articles, but don't stop there. Find a way to understand how you and your organization fit into the overall scheme. Understand what you may need and what you may contribute. Take an honest inventory.

As a nation, we collectively got caught somewhat flat-footed by SARS-CoV-2 (COVID-19). We are most likely better situated to handle the rise—at least for now—in July compared to where we were in March and April of 2020. Some of that is by extreme concerted effort, and some is by luck. A big part is that we were able to make some general improvements in reserve capability (at an enormous financial cost). However, we are a long way from addressing the original concerns we had that led to our extreme lack of reserve to respond initially. Our only real countermeasure in the earlier months of 2020 was to shut down society as we understood it in an attempt to give hospitals a chance to catch up. We transferred to lack of reserve problem of hospitals to the country at large, which was not unreasonable at that time. Some people had the reserves to handle the consequences of that strategy; some did not. Lives have been inexorably altered. We as a health care system need to find a way to be better prepared to handle all-cause hazards that our communities may require. If not because it is the right thing for us to do, then because we need viable communities as much as they need us. In fact, we are one and the same thing. Good luck and stay well. Thanks for all that you do.

Ronald F. Martin, MD, FACS
Kalispell Regional Healthcare
Kalispell Regional Medical Group
Division of HPB Surgery and Surgical Oncology
310 Sunnyview Lane
Kalispell, MT 59901, USA

E-mail address:
rfmcescna@gmail.com

Preface

Rural Surgery: Then, Now, and Beyond

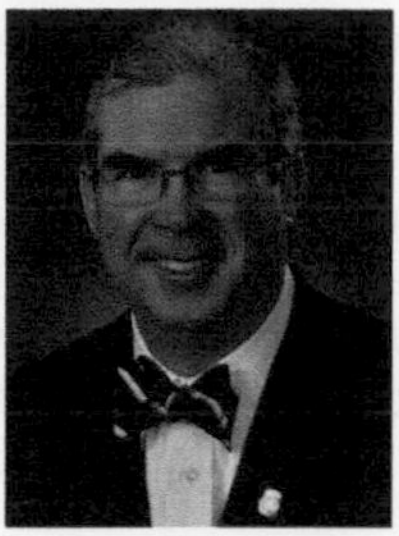

Tyler G. Hughes, MD, FACS
Editor

This issue of *Surgical Clinics* was in the process of editing when the great pandemic of 2020 swept over the world. As of this writing, how the events of that historic event will change the practice of surgery in multiple venues remains enigmatic. Osler wisely said, "In order to solve a problem one must first understand the problem." Knowing the prime issues of rural surgery before the pandemic without doubt is part of understanding its problems and future.

While the venue in which surgery is practiced varies, the goal of operating remains unchanged: to perform at one's highest level to treat the sick and injured. The problem of how to provide the best care for a patient regardless of place is more pressing than ever in rural surgery today. In the United States, the training paradigm for surgeons still reflects the demographic of the times in which it was developed. The Halstedian model of training was developed in an agrarian nation just coming into the industrial age. During the first two-thirds of the twentieth century, the world in general and the United States in particular became a much more urbanized and industrial economy. As these changes altered the environment in which surgery was practiced, a natural process of specialization has changed the role of the general surgeon.

The infrastructure of medicine as well as its payment system radically changed over the twentieth century, and such changes continue in the twenty-first century. Most of the hospitals in existence for surgeons practicing in rural areas were founded post-World War II. These general hospitals were meant to supply a full continuum of care to a community, and surgical services were largely provided by surgeons working independently of the hospital itself.

By the dawn of the first decade of the twenty-first century, the previously adequate solutions were becoming out-of-date. Visionaries in surgical leadership, like J. David Richardson, Brent Eastman, and Patricia Numann, accurately identified these shortcomings and connected with their rural counterparts to pursue solutions for a new

Surg Clin N Am 100 (2020) xvii–xviii
https://doi.org/10.1016/j.suc.2020.06.007
0039-6109/20/© 2020 Published by Elsevier Inc.

era. The results of their leadership can be seen on the pages herein. For the last 20 years, there has been an increasing movement to face the moral imperative of providing high-quality surgical care to the vast regions of the world that are rural. Close to 40% of the world's population live in rural or austere environments. As urban medicine advances in its application of technology and sophisticated big data-driven evidence, the rural world must find ways to provide the best care closest to home for their teeming masses, which are older, sicker, and less well funded than their urban cohorts.

This journal is yet another iteration of this movement, addressing the needs unique to rural surgery along with solutions being developed by those in major medical centers and isolated rural locations. In this issue, we discuss the real economic issues causing loss of surgical access, the demographics of the changing rural population (demographics are destiny), the scope of practice of the modern rural surgeon, the training challenges for those going into this "new" specialty, tools for research that apply to rural surgery, the status of the rural surgery workforce, patient-transfer issues, developing substantive quality improvement processes even in the smallest of facilities, and much more.

The medical and economic events caused by the pandemic have further exposed the critical nature and differences between care delivery in a rural versus urban environment. In these pages, you will find some of those reasons and an understanding of the problem overall, which existed before and will persist after the coronavirus becomes part of the history of medicine in the twenty-first century.

I am expressly grateful to each of the authors, each of whom is a true expert living and working in the rural world. There are great obstacles ahead for rural surgery. In these pages, we continue the work of solving what at times feels like impossible problems. After all, isn't that the *raison d'être* of surgery in all venues?

Tyler G. Hughes, MD, FACS
University of Kansas School of Medicine
Salina Campus
138 North Santa Fe Avenue
Salina, KS 67601, USA

E-mail address:
Thughes55@kumc.edu

Demographics in Rural Populations

Jarron M. Saint Onge, PhD[a,b,*], Sarah Smith, MA[a]

KEYWORDS

• Rural health • Population trends • Demographics • Population health
• Social determinants of health • Age structure • Health disparities • Rural poverty

KEY POINTS

- Rural population trends include depopulation, aging, and increasing race/ethnic diversity in addition to lower socioeconomic status and ongoing health concerns.
- An understanding of rural health requires a focus on both compositional and contextual concepts of rurality.
- Changing population trends have implications for cultural norms, health opportunities, health complications, and postoperative care.
- Rural health needs to move beyond health care to consider how broader sociodemographic factors influence patient profiles and successful health outcomes.

INTRODUCTION

Rural health care policy has become an important component of US health policy, but additional work needs to be done in addressing rural population health needs. Although access to quality health care providers and timely services remains an ongoing rural health priority,[1,2] rural surgeons can benefit further from information about the underlying social conditions and broad structural factors that continue to put rural residents at a health disadvantage. A demographic approach presents an opportunity to consider the role of population demographics in current and future health care. Accordingly, the goal of this article is 3-fold: to describe current rural demographic trends, to consider how these trends are related to patient populations, and to consider implications specific to rural health care and surgery. By highlighting demographic trends in rural areas, considerations are offered for future innovations in rural health practices.

[a] Department of Sociology, University of Kansas, 716 Fraser Hall 1415 Jayhawk Boulevard, Lawrence, KS 66045, USA; [b] Department of Population Health, University of Kansas Medical Center, Kansas City, KS, USA
* Corresponding author.
E-mail address: jsaintonge@ku.eu

Surg Clin N Am 100 (2020) 823–833
https://doi.org/10.1016/j.suc.2020.06.005
surgical.theclinics.com
0039-6109/20/

ROLE OF DEMOGRAPHY

Demography is the systematic study of the size and composition of populations. As explored more fully in this issue, rural demographics continue to have an impact on the rural workforce (see J. Patrick Walker's article, "Status of the Rural Surgical Workforce," in this issue) and the operating environment for rural hospital and clinic success. Yet, changes in populations resulting from birth, deaths, and migration also have consequences for the age, sex, and racial/ethnic distributions of a population as well as subsequent health conditions. A demographic perspective recognizes how individuals are embedded within populations and history and aims to move beyond epidemiologic description to understand why a population is healthy or unhealthy.[3] A clearer understanding of rural demographic processes allows both surgeons and administrators the opportunity to better plan and to more clearly grasp current issues facing patient populations and population health.

RURAL DEFINITIONS

Assumptions about what it means to be "rural" often are misinformed and taken for granted. Geographic definitions remain subject to scrutiny depending on the aims or goals of the institutions using the definitions. For example, US Census Bureau rural definitions are based primarily on population size and density, whereas rural areas also may be defined by rural-urban commuting area codes, by Rural-Urban Continuum Codes, or as Office of Management and Budget nonmetropolitan regions. Although the various codes are nearly identical when simply distinguishing between urban and rural, key differences emerge when disaggregating into more specific categories. A single rural category fails to distinguish between small rural areas, more populated rural destinations, and frontier areas, particularly when determined at the county level. Importantly, these debates go beyond mere academic discussions, where research has shown mortality disparities across multiple rural classifications,[4] and funding opportunities based on rural inclusion criteria have implications for planning and development of health care resources.[5]

MEANING OF PLACE

Demography offers both theoretic and empirical tools to contextualize regional similarities of rural populations, while recognizing the health implications of their unique differences. Although frequently treated as a homogeneous category, rural America comprises diverse and heterogenous populations. For instance, the rural South or the Mississippi delta are quite different in both race/ethnicity and socioeconomic status (SES) compared with the rural Midwest or rural border counties.

An understanding of rural demographics must begin with a conceptualization of place. Conceptualizing the effects of "rural" as a place has multiple meanings, where it includes both the compositional effects (ie, proportion of people in an area with certain individual characteristics) and the contextual effects (ie, opportunities or infrastructural resources in an area). Both need to be considered when examining population health trends.

Compositional effects refer to characteristics of a population. For example, understanding the relative proportion of the population not in the labor force compared with the working age population (ie, dependency ratio) has implications for local tax shortages or health care consumption patterns. Contextual effects refer to the unique aspects of rural areas above and beyond the composition of the local populations. Contextual effects can be disaggregated further into opportunity structures or sociocultural features of an area.[6] For example, opportunity structures include access to material resources, such as health care, but also access to clean air, stable housing, and safe working spaces. Sociocultural factors include factors linked to regional history and culture, such as health-related norms, shared values, access to social networks, and collective efficacy.

Although population shifts frequently are interpreted in terms of compositional changes (eg, more poorer individuals in an area), these also should be more attention given to the harder to measure contextual factors. For example, a low-income, low-educated population (ie, compositional) also may live in an area with strong religious ties that include health-promoting norms and social sanctions (ie, contextual) that promote well-being.

POPULATION DATA

Data on population demographics are readily available for analysis and can be utilized for both local and regional areas. The US Census provides easy public access to population data at data.census.gov to analyze local-level demographic trends. As an example, this article presents data from the 2014 to 2018 American Community Survey (ACS) 5-year estimates, a nationwide survey that provides communities with demographic data. The 5-year file of the ACS is designed to provide data at smaller levels of geography (eg, counties). Population pyramids are presented, a simple demographic technique to visually compare population trends by urban and rural counties in the United States to demonstrate how population data can be used to understand trends relevant to rural surgeons.

The ACS data were matched with Economic Research Service Rural-Urban Continuum Codes to identify counties as either metropolitan or nonmetropolitan areas. The authors disaggregated urban and rural areas by sex and age, to describe general US population trends and differences between urban and rural areas. **Fig. 1** shows population pyramids by urban and rural areas, with the bars representing the percentage of the overall total in each age category.

These data are indicative of multiple trends in rural populations. First, comparisons of the population pyramids show slightly lower proportions of the overall populations in the youngest age categories, indicating an aging population. The slightly smaller rural populations in lower age categories suggest lower rates of childbirth and populations that consequently are less likely to replace their populations through childbirth. Second, the rural population is top-heavier, beginning with individuals aged 55 and older. Although the 45-to-54 age group is nearly identical to urban populations, higher

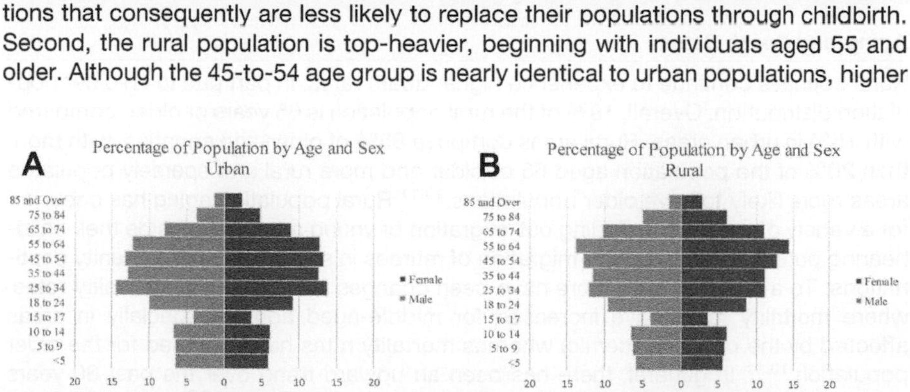

Fig. 1. Population periods of 2014 to 2018 US urban (A) and rural (B) populations. (*Data from* United States Census Bureau. American community survey 2014-2018 5-year estimates. Available at: https://www.census.gov/newsroom/press-releases/2019/acs-5-year.html. Accessed February 1, 2020.)

differences are found in both the 55-to-64 (approximately 1%) and 64-to-74 (approximately 2%) age categories. Third, a higher proportion of women in the older age categories is found in both rural and urban areas. The rural-urban sex differences become more pronounced in the 75-and-over age groups, where there are more aging rural women, presumably due to higher mortality rates among rural men. The fourth trend of note is the working age population differences in the 25-to-44 populations, representing approximately 27% versus 22% of the total urban and rural population, respectively.

Taken together, population pyramids demonstrate the usefulness of identifying population trends. These are useful particularly at a more local, county level. Accordingly, these population distributions are related to community-level demands and needs for goods and services, consumption patterns, and specific health care needs. Health facility size and services rely on both the population size and composition as well as the availability of resources to pay for these services.

RURAL TRENDS

Demography offers several insights for population health and rural surgery. Rural America currently is characterized by 3 recent demographic trends, including depopulation, increasing death rates, and increasing diversity.[7,8] Additionally, descriptions of SES and health trends provide further information for ongoing rural health needs.

Depopulation

Depopulation, or the loss of population, is of ongoing concern for health care facilities, the rural workforce, and substantive tax bases. In previous years, out-migration and depopulation were offset by higher fertility rates in rural regions, particularly by immigrant populations. And although some rural areas have seen net population gains, this is limited mostly to rural areas with greater population density, scenic qualities, or locations near major cities and presents new challenges for long-term residents who often fail to economically benefit.[9] Beginning in 2010, US rural counties began experiencing net population loss with more loss experienced in more remote rural areas.[10] Chronic out-migration has direct impacts on population size but also is related to both fertility and mortality that continue to exacerbate population loss, with fewer young people to have children and an aging population with more deaths.[8]

Aging and Death Rates

Rural counties continue to experience higher death rates, in part due to an older population distribution. Overall, 19% of the rural population is 65 years or older, compared with 15% in urban areas. Rural areas comprise 85% of older-age counties, with more than 20% of the population aged 65 or older and more rural and sparsely populated areas more likely to have older populations.[10,11] Rural population aging has occurred for a variety of reasons, including out-migration of young adults (alongside their child-bearing potential) and some in-migration of retirees in scenic and high-amenity destinations. To a lesser extent, there have been changes in age-specific mortality rates, where mortality rates have increased for middle-aged adults (especially in areas affected by the opioid epidemic) whereas mortality rates have declined for the older population.[10,11] In general, there has been an upward trend over the past 30 years in the number of counties experiencing more deaths than births,[12] which continues to have an impact on the depopulation of rural communities.

Rural residents generally have higher rates of disease, more disability, and lower life expectancies. Overall, urban life expectancy has continued to increase, whereas rural life expectancy has stagnated over the past decades. The rural-urban gap in life expectancy increased from a 0.4-year disadvantage between 1969 and 1971 to 2.0 years between 2005 and 2009.[13] Compared with urban areas, rural areas tend to have both higher rates of all-cause mortality and cause-specific mortality disparities.[14,15] These rural disadvantages are larger for minorities, with non-Hispanic blacks, and Native Americans/Alaskan Indians demonstrating gaps of approximately 10 years compared with metropolitan-residing whites or Asians.[13]

Racial/Ethnic Diversity

Rural areas in the United States are less racially and ethnically diverse than metropolitan areas. In 2017, racial/ethnic minorities comprised 22% of the rural population compared with 42% of the urban population.[10] Rural areas, however, are becoming more diverse over time. The rural population in 2017 was approximately 80% non-Hispanic white, 9% Hispanic, 8% black, 2% American Indian, and 1% Asian. The population of racial/ethnic minorities in nonmetropolitan areas increased approximately 20% between 2000 and 2010, whereas the rural non-Hispanic white population exhibited negligible growth during this period.[16] In particular, the rural Hispanic population grew by 45%, accounting for 56% of all nonmetropolitan population growth during this period.[16]

The relative growth of the rural Hispanic population is attributable to the relatively young age structure among this population, creating a surplus of births over deaths, whereas mortality diminishes the numbers of the aging white population.[7] Hispanic growth in rural areas, however, is spatially concentrated, with less than 10% of nonmetropolitan counties accounting for 50% of Hispanic population growth.[16]

Rural America, once an image of ethnic homogeneity, now is considered a new immigrant destination area. This is linked to growth in low-wage industries, such as manufacturing, construction, and meatpacking, where jobs are "difficult, dirty, and sometimes dangerous" and often shunned by native-born workers.[17] More than two-thirds of rural immigrants are undocumented.[18] Immigrants to nonmetropolitan areas tend to be young and of childbearing age with high fertility rates.[19] Rural immigrants are less fluent in English, less educated, and more likely to be undocumented compared with previous generations.[18] Although immigration in rural areas can halt the negative social and economic consequences of depopulation and produce diverse, integrated rural communities, it also can result in divisive rhetoric and segregation and undermine community social cohesion.[20] As a result, the impacts of rural immigration and growing diversity on rural health and health care may depend largely on the social and policy context of the area.

Socioeconomic Status

Rural areas consistently have been associated with low levels of SES, including income, education, and occupational prestige. In the past few decades, rural communities have experienced structural and economic transformations that have increased both poverty and inequality.[21] In 2017, the rural poverty rate was 16.4% compared with 12.9% for urban areas.[22] Between 2000 and 2017, poverty rates declined across the United States, but urban poverty rates declined at a higher rate than in rural areas.[22] Among rural areas, poverty rates are highest in more remote and rural counties. Additionally, the rural poor tend to be spatially concentrated, geographically isolated, socially disorganized, and, in many instances, also race/ethnically concentrated, increasingly referred to as rural ghettos.[23–25]

Rural areas differ substantially from urban areas in educational attainment. Although the share of the rural population with less than a high school education has declined to

15% (compared with 13% in urban areas), there remains a large and growing rural-urban gap in the proportion of the population with a bachelor's degree or higher. In 2015, only 19% of rural residents had a bachelor's degree or higher compared with 33% of the urban population.[26] Rural-urban educational disparities are attributable to out-migration, where higher returns to education are found in urban areas in both earnings and employment.

Rural educational attainment also varies substantially by race, with 24% of blacks and 39% of Hispanics having less than a high school diploma, with both of these groups less than half as likely as whites to have a bachelor's degree or higher. Low education and poverty rates are highly correlated in rural counties, and both poverty and low educational attainment are concentrated particularly in the rural South and Appalachia.[26]

As the rural population has gotten older, labor force participation has been reduced dramatically in rural regions. Although urban and rural unemployment rates have declined at similar rates since the Great Recession, rural areas have lagged considerably behind urban areas in increases in employment rates over this period. Between 2010 and 2018, rural employment grew 0.4% annually compared with 1.5% in metro areas.[22] Falling unemployment accompanied by slow employment growth in rural areas is attributable to relatively low labor force participation due to aging, lower levels of education, and higher rates of disability alongside low rural population growth.

IMPLICATIONS AND CHALLENGES

The challenges facing rural health care and rural surgery in part reflect the characteristics of each individual local area. Yet, there are general challenges faced across all rural regions. The often-cited phrase, "demography is destiny," is both an ongoing challenge and an opportunity for improvement, where an understanding of demographic trends has the potential for important policy and practice investments. Several overlapping trends with implications for rural health and health care related to rural surgery are highlighted.

Health Care Access

Several direct factors put rural residents at risk of negative health outcomes, with access to quality services and providers frequently listed among major concerns.[1] In terms of resources, there remain challenges in recruiting and retaining high-quality health professionals. Areas characterized by long-term outmigration and population decline are less desirable to highly educated health specialists and surgeons due to variety of population-related issues, such as limited marriage markets, low-quality schools, and a lack of other urban amenities (eg, funding for arts). New innovations and recent initiatives have begun to demonstrate the potential of telemedicine and urban-rural partnerships to partially address the health care needs of areas with low access to services and providers.

Even when facilities and staffing are in place, rural residents may continue to require assistance in gaining access to care. Compared with urban residents, rural residents have limited access to employer-sponsored health insurance. Also, physical and social barriers limit the odds of rural residents enrolling in government programs, such as Medicaid. Attempts to meet health care needs among this population may need to go beyond government expansions of safety net programs, because unmet needs and limited preventive care often lead to severe and complicated health care needs.

Social Determinants of Health

Although timely health care access remains critical to address acute conditions, such as heart attacks or strokes, additional attention must be given to the social conditions that continue to put rural residents at elevated risk for poor health conditions in the first place. As described previously, rural communities experience many social disadvantages. Key social determinants of health, such as SES, are linked to contextual factors, such as social connections, opportunities for health promoting activities, and psychosocial issues, including social isolation or regional stressors. Attention to these determinants through safeguards or material resources has the potential to limit environmental exposures, influence health norms, reduce the incidence of negative health behaviors, and increase the knowledge and opportunities to reduce potential health complications.

Health Behaviors

Health behaviors do not occur in isolation and tend to comprise health behavior lifestyles that reflect both sociodemographic and cultural factors.[27,28] Rural health behaviors include a higher prevalence of smoking, lower likelihoods of meeting physical activity recommendations, high rates of obesity, low fiber and fruit intake, and higher intake of sweetened beverages.[29,30] Rural residents experience contextual factors that limit their ability to enact healthy lifestyles, including built environments that are not conducive to physical activity, limited access to healthy food, and health-compromising norms. Yet, efforts are beginning to demonstrate how primary health providers can partner with local facilities to increase healthy lifestyles in rural areas.[31,32]

Substance Use and Behavioral Health

Rural regions have high rates of unmet mental illness needs with implications for substance use issues. High prevalence of depression and substance use are a problem in rural areas as well as high rates of suicide mortality.[33,34] Rural areas have limited drug prevention and treatment programs.[35] Rural health care providers need to address chronic behavioral health issues, normative resistance to treatment, and ongoing efforts to manage pain in lieu of potential addictions.

Occupational Hazards

Rural residents have up to 35% higher nonfatal injury hospitalization rates compared with urban residents, along with nearly twice the injury mortality rate.[36,37] This is due to both structural and cultural factors. For example, rural residents are at much greater risk of motor vehicle injuries due to in part both reckless driving and a lack of crash reduction features on rural highways. Rural residents also are more likely to be engaged in some of the most dangerous occupations, such as mining and agriculture, and experience high numbers of work-related injuries.[37] Although preventive and safety measures can be put into place, additional concerns to address cultural norms also are needed to reduce risky behaviors, particularly among rural men in dangerous occupations.

Health Literacy and Cultural Health Capital

The relatively low SES and growing immigrant populations in rural areas suggests that to reduce health disparities and improve rural health, health care workers and rural surgeons must be attuned to issues of both health literacy and cultural health capital, "a specialized form of cultural capital that can be leveraged in health care contexts to effectively engage with medical providers."[38] Cultural health capital includes elements, such as medical knowledge and vocabulary, the ability to efficiently communicate information with providers, and a proactive stance toward health. Low SES and immigrant populations are disproportionately likely to lack cultural health capital, creating disadvantages or perceived noncompliance in health care interactions.

Social Support and Social Capital

Older rural residents are more likely than their urban counterparts to have a spouse and a larger number of children on average, but they also are more likely to have greater geographic distance between them and their adult children.[39] Follow-up medical care and barriers to transportation require heightened consideration of social support and home environments. An aging population requires more consistent assistance from caregivers. Out-migration, particularly among children, also may put older rural residents at risk of social isolation and depression. Although rural communities have long been characterized by high levels of social cohesion and social networks (particularly through religious organizations), changing demographics have left an aging, non-Hispanic white population increasingly isolated in socially and culturally contested spaces.[40]

Veterans

A disproportionate number of US military veterans reside in rural regions, with veterans more likely to both originate from and return to rural areas.[41] Although the veteran population is expected to decrease over time, the median age will continue to increase along with more rural concentration. In general, veterans have higher prevalence rates of diagnosed health conditions, such as cancer, chronic obstructive pulmonary disease, and diabetes.[41] Health care planning for veterans is challenging particularly because most veterans have multiple sources of health coverage and rely on a variety of providers for multiple conditions. Communities would benefit from a further understanding of veteran needs and opportunities to work with Veterans Administration (VA) facilities. Ongoing shifts in service-related disabilities and VA eligibility requirements will continue to have future implications on both local VA and civilian health care.

Children

Although a majority of rural health research is focused on adults, rural children's health also should be noted. Compared with urban residents, rural children are at increased risk of obesity, higher prevalence of dental issues, infectious diseases, and alcohol and drug use. In part, this likely is due to both material resources and social factors, such as unique rural norms and culture that have an impact on both risk and resiliency factors.[42]

Vulnerable Populations

Compared with rural whites, rural minorities have worse health, with American Indians and Alaska Natives having the highest mortality rates among the rural poor.[43] Although many rural American Indians/Alaska Natives receive services through the Indian Health Service (IHS), the IHS is not a comprehensive source of health insurance and lacks sufficient funding to ensure access to health care for this population.[44] In addition to issues of access to care, the American Indian/Alaska Native population suffers from high rates of poverty, low levels of education, and cultural differences and discrimination in health care. Substance use and mental illness are other major concerns among this population, with more than 6 times the alcohol-induced mortality rate and 1.7 times the suicide rate relative to the overall population.[45]

Rural sexual minority (eg, lesbian, gay, bisexual, and transgender [LGBT+]) populations also face disparities in health and health care. The rural LGBT+ population is at greater risk for substance use and depression and faces issues of stigma both in the community and in health care interactions. Additional barriers include provider knowledge, attitudes, and sensitivity and lack of access to LGBT+-friendly providers in rural areas.[46]

SUMMARY

Population health is inherently the result of demographic processes. Insights into local health issues and solutions to concerns in health care can benefit from clear, meaningful definitions, and understandings of rural population dynamics. Population declines, migration, aging, and socioeconomic and racial diversity of rural communities continue to challenge local institutions. Solutions need to move beyond health care, to determine how local government, schools, and labor market decisions can work together to address both push and pull factors for migrants and meet the health needs of the population. Changing demographics also present opportunities for innovation. In-migration of new residents that differ in age and ethnic diversity brings unique social resources and ingenuity that may benefit the health care system in particular ways through new behaviors and social norms that influence health behaviors.

A demographic perspective offers potential insights into the practice of rural health care. Rather than focusing simply on individual epidemiologic risk factors, a demographic approach on population distributions incorporates both compositional and contextual explanations and identifies how trends in socioeconomic and sociodemographic characteristics can influence health and heath care.

REFERENCES

1. Bolin JN, Bellamy GR, Ferdinand AO, et al. Rural healthy people 2020: new decade, same challenges. J Rural Health 2015;31(3):326–33.
2. Douthit N, Kiv S, Dwolatzky T, et al. Exposing some important barriers to health care access in the rural USA. Public Health 2015;129(6):611–20.
3. Berkman LF, Kawachi I. A historical framework for social inequality. In: Berkman LF, Kawachi I, editors. Social epidemiology. New York: Oxford University Press; 2000. p. 3–10.
4. James WL. All rural places are not created equal: revisiting the rural mortality penalty in the United States. Am J Public Health 2014;104(11):2122–9.
5. Bennett KJ, Borders TF, Holmes GM, et al. What is rural? Challenges and implications of definitions that inadequately encompass rural people and places. Health Aff 2019;38(12):1985–92.
6. Macintyre S, Ellaway A, Cummins S. Place effects on health: how can we conceptualise, operationalise and measure them? Soc Sci Med 2002;55(1):125–39.
7. Johnson KM, Lichter DT. Diverging demography: hispanic and non-hispanic contributions to U.S. population redistribution and diversity. Popul Res Policy Rev 2016;35(5):705–25.
8. Johnson KM, Lichter DT. Rural depopulation: growth and decline processes over the past century. Rural Sociol 2019;84(1):3–27.

9. Saint Onge JM, Hunter LM, Boardman JD. Population growth in high-amenity rural areas: does it bring socioeconomic benefits for long-term residents? Soc Sci Q 2007;88(2):366–81.
10. Cromartie J. Rural America at a glance. 2018th edition. Washington, DC: US Department of Agriculture. Economic Research Bulletin; 2018. p. 200.
11. Glasgow N, Brown DL. Rural ageing in the United States: trends and contexts. J Rural Stud 2012;28(4):422–31.
12. Johnson KM. Deaths exceed births in record number of U.S. counties. Durham (NH): Carsey Institute, University of New Hamshire; 2013. p. 1–2. Vol Fact Sheet No. 25.
13. Singh GK, Siahpush M. Widening rural–urban disparities in life expectancy, US, 1969–2009. Am J Prev Med 2014;46(2):e19–29.
14. Cossman JS, James WL, Cosby AG, et al. Underlying causes of the emerging nonmetropolitan mortality penalty. Am J Public Health 2010;100(8):1417–9.
15. Roth AR, Denney JT, Amiri S, et al. Characteristics of place and the rural disadvantage in deaths from highly preventable causes. Soc Sci Med 2020;245: 112689.
16. Lichter DT. Immigration and the new racial diversity in rural America. Rural Sociol 2012;77(1):3–35.
17. Massey DS, editor. New faces in new places: the changing geography of American immigration. New York: Russell Sage Foundation; 2008.
18. Farmer FL, Moon ZK. An empirical examination of characteristics of mexican migrants to metropolitan and nonmetropolitan areas of the United States. Rural Sociol 2009;74(2):220–40.
19. Lichter DT, Johnson KM, Turner RN, et al. Hispanic assimilation and fertility in new destinations. Int Migr Rev 2012;46(4):767–91.
20. Carr PJ, MacDonald J, Sampson RJ, et al. Can immigration save small-town America? Hispanic boomtowns and the uneasy path to renewal. Ann Am Acad Pol Soc Sci 2012;641(1):38–57.
21. Albrecht DE, Albrecht SL. Poverty in nonmetropolitan America: impacts of industrial, employment, and family structure variables. Rural Sociol 2000;65(1):87–103.
22. Pender J, Hertz T, Cromartie J, et al. Rural America at a glance. 2019th edition. Washington, DC: US Department of Agriculture. Economic Information Bulletin; 2019. p. 212.
23. Lichter DT, Parisi D, Taquino MC, et al. Residential segregation in new Hispanic destinations: cities, suburbs, and rural communities compared. Soc Sci Res 2010;39(2):215–30.
24. Moller S, Alderson AS, Nielsen F. Changing patterns of income inequality in US counties, 1970–2000. Am J Sociol 2009;114(4):1037–101.
25. Burton LM, Lichter DT, Baker RS, et al. Inequality, family processes, and health in the "new" rural America. Am Behav Sci 2013;57(8):1128–51.
26. Marre A. Rural education at a glance. 2017th edition. Washington, DC: US Department of Agriculture. Economic Information Bulletin; 2017. p. 171.
27. Saint Onge JM, Krueger PM. Health lifestyle behaviors among US adults. SSM Popul Health 2017;3:89–98.
28. Saint Onge JM, Krueger PM. Education and racial-ethnic differences in types of exercise in the United States. J Health Soc Behav 2011;52(2):197–211.
29. Matthews KA, Croft JB, Liu Y, et al. Health-related behaviors by urban-rural county classification — United States, 2013. MMWR Surveill Summ 2017; 66(5):1–8.

30. Trivedi T, Liu J, Probst J, et al. Obesity and obesity-related behaviors among rural and urban adults in the USA. Rural Remote Health 2015;15(4):3267.
31. Befort CA, VanWormer JJ, DeSouza C, et al. Protocol for the rural engagement in primary care for optimizing weight reduction (RE-POWER) trial: comparing three obesity treatment models in rural primary care. Contemp Clin Trials 2016;47: 304–14.
32. Vadheim LM, Brewer KA, Kassner DR, et al. Effectiveness of a lifestyle intervention program among persons at high risk for cardiovascular disease and diabetes in a rural community. J Rural Health 2010;26(3):266–72.
33. Borders TF, Booth BM. Rural, suburban, and urban variations in alcohol consumption in the United States: findings from the National Epidemiologic Survey on Alcohol and Related Conditions. J Rural Health 2007;23(4):314–21.
34. Simmons LA, Braun B, Charnigo R, et al. Depression and poverty among rural women: a relationship of social causation or social selection? J Rural Health 2008;24(3):292–8.
35. Gamm L, Stone S, Pittman S. Mental health and mental disorders – a rural challenge. In: Gamm L, Hutchison L, Dabney B, et al, editors. Rural Healthy People 2010: A Companion Document to Healthy People 2010, Vol. 1. College Station, TX: Texas A&M University System Health Science Center, School of Rural Public Health, Southwest Rural Health Research Center; 2003. p. 165–70.
36. Coben JH, Tiesman HM, Bossarte RM, et al. Rural-urban differences in injury hospitalizations in the U.S., 2004. Am J Prev Med 2009;36(1):49–55.
37. Peek-Asa C, Zwerling C, Stallones L. Acute traumatic injuries in rural populations. Am J Public Health 2004;94(10):1689–93.
38. Shim JK. Cultural health capital: a theoretical approach to understanding health care interactions and the dynamics of unequal treatment. J Health Soc Behav 2010;51(1):1–15.
39. Glasgow N. Rural/urban patterns of aging and caregiving in the United States. J Fam Issues 2000;21(5):611–31.
40. Skinner MW, Winterton R. Interrogating the contested spaces of rural aging: implications for research, policy, and practice. Gerontologist 2017;58(1):15–25.
41. Eibner C, Krull H, Brown KM, et al. Current and projected characteristics and unique health care needs of the patient population served by the department of veterans affairs. Rand Health Q 2016;5(4):13.
42. Pettigrew J, Miller-Day M, Krieger J, et al. The rural context of illicit substance offers: a study of Appalachian rural adolescents. J Adolesc Res 2012;27(4): 523–50.
43. Baldwin L-M, Grossman DC, Casey S, et al. Perinatal and infant health among rural and urban American Indians/Alaska Natives. Am J Public Health 2002;92(9): 1491–7.
44. Warne D, Frizzell LB. American Indian health policy: historical trends and contemporary issues. Am J Public Health 2014;104(Suppl 3):S263–7.
45. Indian Health Service. Indian Health Disparities. 2019. Available at: https://www.ihs.gov/sites/newsroom/themes/responsive2017/display_objects/documents/factsheets/Disparities.pdf. Accessed December 20, 2019.
46. Rosenkrantz DE, Black WW, Abreu RL, et al. Health and health care of rural sexual and gender minorities: a systematic review. Stigma Health 2017;2(3): 229–43.

Rural Surgery and Status of the Rural Workplace

Hospital Survival and Economics

Adrian Diaz, MD, MPH[a,b,c], Timothy M. Pawlik, MD, MPH, MTS, PhD[c,*]

KEYWORDS

• Rural • Surgery • Access • Hospital closure

KEY POINTS

- One in 5 residents (nearly 60 million people) live in a rural area, accounting for 12% of the 35 million hospitalizations across the United States.
- Since 2005, 162 rural hospitals have closed, and the rate of rural hospital closures seems to be accelerating with an additional 700 hospitals at risk of closure.
- Major drivers of rural hospital closures are poor financial health, aging facilities, and low occupancy rates.
- Rural hospitals are particularly vulnerable to policy and market changes, and even small changes can have a disproportionate effect on rural hospital financial viability.
- Surgery can be safely performed in rural hospitals; however, hospital closures may be putting the rural population at increased risk of morbidity and mortality from surgical disease.

Funding: Dr A. Diaz received salary support from the Veterans' Affairs Office of Academic Affiliations during the time of the study.
Conflicts of interest: The authors have no conflicts of interest to report.
Disclaimer: This article does not necessarily represent the views of the United States government or Department of Veterans' Affairs.
[a] National Clinician Scholars Program at the Institute for Healthcare Policy and Innovation, University of Michigan, 2800 Plymouth Road, North Campus Research Complex, Building 14 Suite G-100, Ann Arbor, MI 48109, USA; [b] Center for Healthcare Outcomes and Policy, University of Michigan, 2800 Plymouth Road, North Campus Research Complex, Building 16, Ann Arbor, MI 48109, USA; [c] Division of Surgical Oncology, The Ohio State University Wexner Medical Center and James Comprehensive Cancer Center, 395 West 12th Avenue, Suite 670, Columbus, OH 43210, USA
* Corresponding author. Department of Surgery, The Ohio State University, Wexner Medical Center, 395 West 12th Avenue, Suite 670, Columbus, OH 43210.
E-mail address: tim.pawlik@osumc.edu

Surg Clin N Am 100 (2020) 835–847
https://doi.org/10.1016/j.suc.2020.05.009 surgical.theclinics.com
0039-6109/20/

THE RURAL POPULATION AND HOSPITAL CLOSURES

Americans face multiple challenges in accessing health care, including insurance status, health literacy, and cost.[1–3] In particular, residents living in rural areas face additional unique challenges accessing health care.[4,5] For example, people living in rural communities have disproportionately adverse health outcomes, including poorer health, greater disability, and higher age-adjusted mortality.[6–8] Importantly, about 1 in 5 residents, nearly 60 million people, live in a rural area.[9] However, 162 rural hospitals have closed since 2005, and the rate of rural hospital closures seems to be accelerating, with an additional 700 hospitals at risk of closure.[10,11] Some closures are strategic decisions that accompany mergers and acquisitions; however, most rural hospital closures result from the inability to remain profitable.[12]

In 2010, rural areas accounted for 12% of the 35 million hospitalizations across the United States.[13] As such, rural hospital closures are a public health emergency. The reasons for this concerning trend are complex and multifactorial, but hospital, market, and financial factors seem to be the major forces driving these trends. Perhaps most alarming is that the rate of rural hospital closures is accelerating. In 2013 and 2014, the number of rural hospital closures was more than twice the number in 2011 and 2012.[11] Based on estimates by Kaufman and colleagues,[11] among the 47 communities served by these closed hospitals, more than 1.7 million people are now at greater risk of negative health and economic hardship because of the loss of local acute care services. Importantly, this trend has not improved because rural hospitals continue to close at a concerning rate.[10] The most obvious consequence of a rural hospital closure is reduced access to hospital care for the population it served. Analysis by the Medicare Payment Advisory Commission noted that about one-third of hospitals that closed since 2013 were more than 20 miles from the next closest hospital.[14] Similar findings have been reported for disease-specific conditions such as surgery, cancer, and obstetrics.[15–19] Furthermore, this decrease in access can increase the risk of bad outcomes for conditions requiring urgent care, including that for high-risk deliveries, trauma, and coronary artery bypass graft surgery.[17,18,20]

Beyond the most obvious threats to acute inpatient hospital care, additional spillover effects are experienced by rural communities. For example, when a hospital closes, access to nonhospital care can also suffer because many specialists cluster around hospitals. In particular, when a rural hospital closes, mental health and substance use care are most likely to be in short supply.[21] Less obvious, but no less concerning, is that a hospital's closure negatively affects the economics of the community it served. When a hospital closes, all the individuals formerly employed by the hospital need to find other jobs. In addition, jobs in related and supporting industries, including food and laundry services and construction, can also be lost. Those losses exert a downward impact on the local economy. As individuals directly affected become unemployed, less revenue is infused into the local economy, threatening the employment of others. All told, when a hospital closes, per capita income in its community declines by 4% and the unemployment rate increases 1.6%, according to data published in *Health Services Research*.[22]

The impact of rural hospital closures is of particular concern because residents of rural communities are typically older and poorer, more dependent on public insurance programs, and in worse health than urban residents.[4,5,8] Policymakers, researchers, and rural residents should be concerned and interested in determining why these hospitals are closing, whether the rate will continue to climb, and what effects there could be on local health care providers and the communities they serve. The reasons for this concerning trend are complex and multifactorial but hospital, market, and financial factors seem to be the major forces driving these trends.

History of Rural Hospital Closures

Although rural hospital closures have been prominent in many recent news stories, these hospital closures are not a new phenomenon.[23] Rural areas have been experiencing hospital closures for decades. Following the Medicare Prospective Payment System for inpatient services implementation in 1983, the risk of negative impact on rural hospitals was identified.[24–26] Concern for the increase of rural hospital closures was enough that the US Health and Human Services Office of the Inspector General published annual updates of hospital closures in the late 1980s and early 1990s.[27] Lillie-Blanton and colleagues[28] were among the first to examine rural and urban closures in the late 1980s and reported that the odds of closure in rural and urban areas differed significantly for private nonprofit hospitals.[25] Subsequently, researchers continued to examine rural hospital closures and noted that, during the 1990s, a total of 460 general hospitals across the United States closed; among these, 35% were located in rural areas.[26] As the rate of hospital closures increased throughout the 1990s, studies consistently found that smaller hospitals were more likely to close, putting rural hospitals at greater risk for closure.[25,29,30]

Concerns about the financial viability of small rural hospitals led to the implementation of the Medicare Rural Hospital Flexibility Program (Flex Program) of 1997, which allows facilities designated as critical access hospitals (CAHs) to be paid on a reasonable cost basis for inpatient and outpatient services.[31] Critical access designation was allowable for hospitals if they had fewer than 25 inpatient beds and were located more than 35 miles away from another hospital.[31] More than 1300 hospitals enrolled in this program, but concern about the resultant Medicare budget growing to more than $9 billion annually led government agencies and advisory groups to call for modification and even elimination of the critical access designation.[32–34] At least 1 study of CAHs found that the Flex Program prevented the closure of many rural hospitals.[30] Advocates for critical access hospitals argue that changes would be disruptive to communities that heavily rely on CAHs for their health care.[35,36]

Factors, New and Old, Associated with Closures

Studies of rural hospital closures have noted that factors can be grouped into 2 main categories: internal hospital factors and external market factors.[29,30,37–44] Internal hospital factors associated with rural hospital closures include poor financial health, aging facilities, low occupancy rates, difficulty recruiting and retaining health professionals, fewer medical services, and a small proportion of outpatient revenue.[29,37,38] An additional source of financial challenge to rural hospitals is shrinking local populations, which means fewer patients to fill beds. To this point, although populations in urban counties have increased since 2000, the census rates of individuals in one-half of rural counties have fallen.[45] Shrinking populations also exacerbate other threats to rural hospital finances. For example, care has been shifting from inpatient to outpatient settings.[11] Although hospitals can and do have outpatient departments, these centers face competition for patients from nonhospital outpatient clinicians and facilities.

External market factors associated with rural hospital closures include socioeconomic factors, including competition. Rural areas tend to have worse population health, higher unemployment rates, and stiffer competition from other hospitals.[46] Hospitals in markets with high proportions of Medicaid or racial and ethnic minority residents, as well as markets with high poverty or uninsured rates, have higher risk of closure.[30,40,41] Measures of competition associated with closure and distress include industry concentration, distance to competitors, and market share.[41–43] Although for-profit hospitals were more likely to close in the past, rates of closures and ownership changes for public facilities may be increasing.[37,38,42] Each of these factors reduces profitability, which is the most consistent predictor of closure and financial distress.[30,39] From 2012 to 2014, rural hospitals averaged a 2% operating margin, compared with 5.9% for urban hospitals.[47] The thinner margins are largely caused by rural hospitals serving populations that tend to have higher rates of chronic illness than those individuals served by urban hospitals.[46] Also, about 60% of rural hospital revenues are from Medicare, Medicaid, or both, compared with 45% for urban hospitals.[48]

Rural hospitals provide patients with the high quality of care while simultaneously tackling challenges caused by their often remote geographic location, small size, limited workforce, and constrained financial resources. The low patient volumes at many rural hospitals make it difficult for these organizations to manage the high fixed costs associated with operating a hospital. In turn, this makes rural hospitals particularly vulnerable to policy and market changes, and to Medicare and Medicaid payment cuts. Even small changes in these programs can have a disproportionate effect on rural hospital financial viability. To this point, in 2013 the Middle Class Tax Relief and Job Creation Act[49] reduced bad debt payments (charity care) to rural hospitals by 35%, and the Budget Control Act of 2011[50] led to a 2% reduction in almost all hospital Medicare payments.

Increasing trends in closures of acute inpatient facilities is a serious but expected outcome at this point in the evolution of the health care system. Potential contributors to the recent increased rate of closures may include the population decrease in rural communities, lower rates of inpatient use, the Affordable Care Act (ACA), as well as other elements of market reform.[11] In an analysis of the increasing rate of rural hospital closures, Kaufamn and colleagues[11] reported that hospitals with higher outpatient, surgery, and obstetric volumes were more likely to be profitable and remain open; hospitals that served communities with a higher percentage of elderly or poor residents were also more likely to have a negative operating margin.

As the rate of closures diminished during the 2000s, attention to the causes and effects of closures decreased. Although cost-based reimbursement may still provide a protective effect, the health care industry is facing a rapidly changing regulatory and economic environment, largely because of the implementation of the ACA. These additional pressures, along with the recent upturn in closure rates, have renewed concern for the viability of rural hospitals in an era of population health, where focus has shifted to value. In particular, the ACA changed the payer mix by increasing the proportion of people with private insurance through the state and federal exchanges. However, some rural communities had only 1 insurer on the exchange. According to a study by the North Carolina Rural Health Research Program, some people bought plans with the cheapest premiums, only to discover that these plans came with unaffordable deductibles and copayments.[51] Furthermore, although some rural hospitals reported decreases in charity care, few reported a positive net financial impact as a result of the ACA's expanded insurance coverage, primarily because respondents thought that bad debt from high-deductible health plans and shortfalls between payments and costs of care in Medicare and Medicaid were growing.

The ACA cuts in Disproportionate Share Hospital (DSH) funding for uncompensated care exacerbated the problem. Under the Patient Protection and Affordable Care Act (PPACA), Medicaid DSH reductions were supposed to go into effect on October 1, 2013.[52] DSH payments go to safety-net hospitals that treat high volumes of poor patients. The PPACA phases out Medicaid DSH payments because the law was supposed to expand Medicaid to all states. However, the Supreme Court ruled that provision was optional for states. The new budget deal delayed all Medicaid DSH cuts until the beginning of fiscal year 2016 and then again to 2020.[53] Downward pressure on reimbursement from Medicare and commercial payers, an increase in high-deductible health plans, below-cost reimbursement for growing numbers of Medicaid enrollees, and anticipated cuts to Medicaid DSH funds all contributed to uncertainty about the long-term financial sustainability of rural hospitals.

The impact of the Medicaid expansion component of the ACA has been mixed. Some evidence shows that states that expanded Medicaid under the ACA were able to reduce the proportion of uncompensated care at rural hospitals; however, the persistence of Medicaid reimbursement at less than cost offset this gain.[54] Although closing hospitals have been more often located in a state not expanding Medicaid, these hospitals are also more likely to be in the South, which historically has lower profitability.[55] Separating the relative importance of these multiple factors is important to understanding the issue, but remains challenging. Nevertheless, rural hospital profit margins have declined in states that did not expand Medicaid, whereas those in most states that did expand Medicaid saw margins remain stable or improve. Specifically, rural hospitals saw an improved chance of turning a profit if located in a state that expanded Medicaid. Across the board, hospitals earned more when located in a state where more people had coverage and saw declines in the level of uncompensated care they gave.[54]

RURAL SURGERY

Surgeons and surgical procedures are essential to the US health care system. Operating room procedures are performed during nearly 30% of all hospital stays.[56] Although rural areas account for about 20% of the population, these hospitals are staffed by only 10% of the physician population.[57] As a consequence, rural patients have less exposure to health care subspecialties, leaving patients to travel long distances to receive therapeutic interventions, often including for surgery.[15,16,58] Further exacerbating the issue, use of surgical procedures is increasing, leading some investigators to suggest that there may be a shortage of surgeons, with the current capacity of medical specialists insufficient for the need.[59–61] To this point, the Association of American Medical Colleges (AAMC) has projected that there will be a physician shortage of roughly 61,700 to 94,700 doctors by 2025.[62] In particular, the AAMC has projected a shortage of surgeons that ranges from 8200 to 24,000. In particular, although certain regions of the country, such as urban centers, have a large number of physicians, rural areas and small cities may have a shortage of doctors.[63]

The decrease in the number of surgeons willing to serve in rural regions also remains a concern.[15,64,65] In turn, any shortage in the surgical workforce is likely to affect underserved areas disproportionally. Although the training of more surgeons may address this problem in part, other initiatives to address surgeon shortages in rural settings are needed. As such, programs to incentivize more surgeons to pursue practice in underserved areas, including rural health care settings, are required.[66] To address the decreasing supply of surgeons in underserved areas, the ACA included a new payment incentive for surgeons who practice and deliver care to patients with limited access to surgical care. Specifically, the ACA called for the Centers for Medicare & Medicaid Services (CMS) to pay a 10% bonus to general surgeons who perform surgical procedures in Health Professional Shortage Areas (Subtitle F, Section 5501).[52] Findings from a single state analysis of this

Medicare Surgery Incentive Payment program reported an associated increase in the number of surgical procedures performed at Health Professional Shortage Area hospitals relative to non–Health Professional Shortage Area hospitals during the incentive period.[67] What remains unknown is whether this incentive payment improved the financial status of rural hospitals or improved the health of the populations being served.

Decreases in access to acute inpatient hospital care can increase the risk of bad outcomes for conditions requiring urgent care, such as trauma and emergency general surgery conditions. In particular, emergency general surgery (EGS) conditions account for more than 2 million hospital admissions in the United States each year.[68] Patients undergoing EGS are more likely to have higher mortality and complication rates compared with similar elective operations.[69] Chaudhary and colleagues[6] suggested that, among EGS patients that are appropriate to treat in rural hospitals, equivalent outcomes are observed between urban and rural hospitals. In contrast, with multidisciplinary surgical care, such as for cancer and cardiac operations, high-volume hospitals have been associated with lower morbidity and mortality compared with low-volume hospitals.[70] These high-volume hospitals are often located in urban areas, which, compounded by the closure of existing rural hospital–based surgical services, may hinder rural community access to high-quality surgical care.[71,72] For example, although the number of hospitals that provided surgical services with an approved American College of Surgeons (ACS) cancer program slightly increased since 2005, the number of people living greater than 60 minutes increased from 6% to 11%.[15] Although the number of major surgical hospitals increased over the decade from 2005 to 2015, there was an 82% increase in the number of people who lived further than an hour from any hospital, let alone a high-volume surgical center.[16] Up to 10% of the United States population resides outside a 48-km (30-mile) radius of a hospital with the capacity to perform adult inpatient surgery.[73]

In a study of surgery in CAHs, Ibrahim and colleagues[74] showed that, among Medicare beneficiaries undergoing common surgical procedures, patients admitted to CAHs versus non–critical access hospitals had no differences in 30-day mortality but had decreased risk-adjusted serious complication rates, and lower adjusted Medicare expenditures, although the patients were less medically complex. In a similar study of a separate cohort of surgical patients, no difference was noted in postoperative mortality, suggesting that CAHs may provide comparable surgical care with their acute care counterparts for general, uncomplicated surgical patients.[75]

These findings may have important policy implications for payers and policy makers responding to mandates in the ACA to evaluate health care services for rural Americans. Patients in rural settings are sometimes reluctant to travel for surgical care, even when told it would lead to a better outcome.[76] These same patients often prefer follow-up locally, independent of where their initial operation occurred. However, recent evidence suggests that patients requiring rehospitalization who are readmitted to the same hospital where they had surgery had improved survival.[77]

THE FUTURE OF RURAL HOSPITALS AND SURGERY

Although understanding the causes of closure in rural hospitals is important, another urgent need is to examine alternative models for the delivery of health services in rural communities. A recent study identified alternative care models used as common strategies following closure of inpatient facilities.[11] These strategies include emergency or urgent care facilities, outpatient centers, and skilled nursing facilities. These models may mitigate the negative impact of hospital closure on rural communities by improving access to health services, providing employment, and reconceiving the rural health paradigm. After the closure of inpatient services, alternative health care delivery models offer the potential to retain local access to some health care services, as well as soften the economic impact of closure on the community. Hospitals are often the largest or the second largest employers in their communities, so the closure of the only hospital in the county can have negative economic effects on a rural community.[22] Although a postclosure health care model may retain some employees, the short-term and long-term economic and health impacts of conversion from inpatient facility to an alternative model have not been explored.

Further knowledge about the financial viability of alternative models would be valuable for hospital administrators considering closure of inpatient facilities. In the wake of closure, these entities are particularly likely to face challenges recruiting providers. Previous studies have found that communities where the hospital has closed have difficulty recruiting and retaining physicians and other providers.[78] Additional challenges may include maximizing value-based payment strategies and retaining market share despite a limited range of services. In addition, it may be beneficial to redesign rural health care policy and reimbursement within a post-ACA environment; for example, improving telehealth payment strategies. A few programs do exist to assist rural hospitals, including the Critical Access Hospital Program[79] and the 340B drug program, which requires pharmaceutical manufacturers to sell drugs at steep discounts to certain hospitals serving larger proportions of low-income and vulnerable people, such as children or patients with cancer.[80] Few programs have squarely focused on addressing the fiscal needs and challenges of rural hospitals and none have been adequate to stem the loss of hospitals in some rural communities.

Recently policy makers are have considered legislative action to preserve access to acute care services in rural areas. As previously described, under Medicare, many rural hospitals are designated as CAHs, meaning these centers have to maintain a certain number of inpatient beds as well as an emergency room. Many hospitals struggle to attract enough inpatients to keep their CAH status. One bill proposed by Senator Grassley (Republican, Iowa), the Rural Emergency Acute Care Hospital Act, S. 1648, would create a new Rural Emergency Hospital classification under Medicare.[81] In this bill, the hospital would have been allowed to have an emergency room and outpatient services, but CAHs would not have to maintain inpatient beds. Alternatively, Representative Graves (Republican, Missouri) proposed the Save Rural Hospital Act, H.R. 2957. Under this bill, titles XVIII of the Social Security Act would have been amended to increase payments to, and modify various requirements regarding, rural health care providers under the Medicare program.[82] However, both of these bills died in congress in 2017.[83,84] Most recently, the CMS finalized a rule in which it will increase the wage index for hospitals with a wage index value below the 25th percentile. CMS are also finalizing changes to the wage index so-called rural floor that will remove urban to rural hospital reclassifications from the calculation of the rural floor wage index value beginning in 2020.[85] These changes by CMS are seen as an aid to rural hospitals; however, to pay for the wage index increase, CMS is using a budget neutrality adjustment to the standardized amount that is applied across all acute inpatient hospitals; therefore, the wage index increase for rural hospitals comes at the expense of urban hospitals.

As the demographics of the country continue to evolve, it is almost certain that rural hospitals will face the most serious challenges in taking care of a disproportionately older, poorer, sicker population. Furthermore, as the nonurban population continues to become smaller, rural hospitals will have to grapple with the challenges of filling empty beds and remaining financially solvent. The trend for increasing alternative health care deliver strategies, including emergency or urgent care facilities, outpatient centers, and ambulatory surgical centers, will undoubtedly play a major role as rural surgical care evolves in the next decade. For urgent and emergent conditions such as trauma and EGS, relationships between rural communities and high-acuity surgical centers must be strengthened so as to disseminate best practices, engage in frictionless knowledge transfer, and (when appropriate) use patient transfers to optimize patient care. In a similar fashion, as complex surgical care continues to centralize, certain parts of the surgical episode (eg, preoperative laboratory tests, postoperative follow-up, adjuvant therapy) should decentralized to local communities. In addition, policy makers and advocates must maintain payment policies that secure safe, local surgical care and allow rural clinicians to accommodate patients locally without increased risk of adverse health care outcomes.

REFERENCES

1. Schoen C, Osborn R, Squires D, et al. Access, affordability, and insurance complexity are often worse in the United States compared to ten other countries. Health Aff (Millwood) 2013;32(12):2205–15.
2. Zogg CK, Scott JW, Jiang W, et al. Differential access to care: The role of age, insurance, and income on race/ethnicity-related disparities in adult perforated appendix admission rates. Surgery 2016;160(5):1145–54.
3. Levy H, Janke A. Health literacy and access to care. J Health Commun 2016; 21(Suppl 1):43–50.
4. Newkirk V. May 29 ADP, 2014. The affordable care Act and insurance coverage in rural areas. Henry J Kais Fam Found; 2014. Available at: https://www.kff.org/uninsured/issue-brief/the-affordable-care-act-and-insurance-coverage-in-rural-areas/. Accessed December 30, 2019.
5. National Rural Health Snapshot. 2010. Available at: https://www.ruralhealthweb.org/about-nrha/about-rural-health-care. Accessed December 30, 2019.
6. Chaudhary MA, Shah AA, Zogg CK, et al. Differences in rural and urban outcomes: a national inspection of emergency general surgery patients. J Surg Res 2017;218:277–84.
7. Comparison of Clinical and Financial Outcomes at Urban and Rural Hospitals among Patients Receiving Inpatient Surgical Care - Journal of the American College of Surgeons. Available at: https://www.journalacs.org/article/S1072-7515(18)30748-8/abstract. Accessed June 13, 2019.
8. Meit M, Knudson A, Gilbert T, et al. The 2014 update of the rural-urban chartbook. 2014. Available at: https://ruralhealth.und.edu/projects/health-reform-policy-research-center/pdf/2014-rural-urban-chartbook-update.pdf. Accessed December 30, 2019.
9. Bureau UC. What is Rural America? The United States Census Bureau. Available at: https://www.census.gov/library/stories/2017/08/rural-america.html. Accessed December 30, 2019.
10. 162 Rural Hospital Closures: January 2005 - Present (120 since 2010). Sheps Center. Available at: https://www.shepscenter.unc.edu/programs-projects/rural-health/rural-hospital-closures/. Accessed December 30, 2019.
11. Kaufman BG, Thomas SR, Randolph RK, et al. The rising rate of rural hospital closures: the rising rate of rural hospital closures. J Rural Health 2016;32(1):35–43.
12. iVantage Health Analytics. Rural Relevance - Vulnerability to Value: A Hospital Strength INDEX Study. Available at: https://www.chartis.com/resources/files/

INDEX_2016_Rural_Relevance_Study_FINAL_Formatted_02_08_16.pdf. Accessed January 4, 2020.
13. Hall MJ, Owings M. Rural and urban hospitals' role in providing inpatient care, 2010. NCHS Data Brief 2014;(147):1–8.
14. Medicare Payment Advisory Commission. Report to the Congress: Medicare and the Health Care Delivery System. 2018. Available at: http://medpac.gov/docs/default-source/reports/jun18_medpacreporttocongress_sec.pdf?sfvrsn=0. Accessed January 4, 2020.
15. Diaz A, Schoenbrunner A, Pawlik TM. Trends in the geospatial distribution of adult inpatient surgical cancer care across the United States. J Gastrointest Surg 2019. https://doi.org/10.1007/s11605-019-04343-5.
16. Diaz A, Schoenbrunner A, Pawlik TM. Trends in the geospatial distribution of inpatient adult surgical services across the United States. Ann Surg 2019. https://doi.org/10.1097/SLA.0000000000003366.
17. Kozhimannil KB, Hung P, Henning-Smith C, et al. Association between loss of hospital-based obstetric services and birth outcomes in rural counties in the United States. JAMA 2018;319(12):1239–47.
18. Hsia RY-J, Shen Y-C. Rising closures of hospital trauma centers disproportionately burden vulnerable populations. Health Aff (Millwood) 2011;30(10):1912–20.
19. Hung P, Henning-Smith CE, Casey MM, et al. Access to obstetric services in rural counties still declining, with 9 percent losing services, 2004–14. Health Aff (Millwood) 2017;36(9):1663–71.
20. Chou S, Deily ME, Li S. Travel distance and health outcomes for scheduled surgery. Med Care 2014;52(3):250–7.
21. Wishner J, Solleveld P, Rudowitz R, et al. A Look at Rural Hospital Closures and Implications for Access to Care. The Kaiser Commission on Medicaid and the Uninsured. Issue Brief July 16. Available at: http://files.kff.org/attachment/issue-brief-a-look-at-rural-hospital-closures-and-implications-for-access-to-care. Accessed December 30, 2019.
22. Holmes GM, Slifkin RT, Randolph RK, et al. The effect of rural hospital closures on community economic health. Health Serv Res 2006;41(2):467–85.
23. A Sense of Alarm as Rural Hospitals Keep Closing - The New York Times. Available at: https://www.nytimes.com/2018/10/29/upshot/a-sense-of-alarm-as-rural-hospitals-keep-closing.html. Accessed January 4, 2020.
24. Rosko MD, Broyles RW. Unintended consequences of prospective payment: erosion of hospital financial position and cost shifting. Health Care Manage Rev 1984;9(3):35–43.
25. Mullner RM, McNeil D. Rural and urban hospital closures: a comparison. Health Aff (Millwood) 1986;5(3):131–41.
26. Mullner RM, Whiteis DS. Rural community hospital closure and health policy. Health Policy 1988;10(2):123–35.
27. Office of Inspector General. Trends in rural hospital Closure: 1987-1991. Available at: https://oig.hhs.gov/oei/reports/oei-04-92-00441.pdf. Accessed January 4, 2020.
28. Lillie-Blanton M, Felt S, Redmon P, et al. Rural and urban hospital closures, 1985-1988: operating and environmental characteristics that affect risk. Inq J Med Care Organ Provis Financ 1992;29:332–44.
29. Chan B, Feldman R, Manning WG. The effects of group size and group economic factors on collaboration: a study of the financial performance of rural hospitals in consortia. Health Serv Res 1999;34(1 Pt 1):9–31.

30. Liu L-L (Sunny), Jervis KJ, Younis M, et al. Hospital financial distress, recovery and closure: Managerial incentives and political costs. J Public Budg Account Financ Manag 2011;23(1):31–68.
31. Medicare Rural Hospital Flexibility Grant Program. Available at: https://www.hrsa.gov/ruralhealth/programopportunities/fundingopportunities/?id=b56d4504-7bf6-4f79-b0e8-37b766f2213e. Accessed December 30, 2019.
32. Congressional Budget Office. Reducing the Deficit: Spending and Revenue Options. Available at: http://www.cbo.gov/sites/default/files/03-10-reducing thedeficit.pdf. Accessed December 30, 2019.
33. Most Critical Access Hospitals Would Not Meet the Location Requirements If Required To Re-enroll in Medicare (OEI-05-12-00080; 08/13). Available at: https://oig.hhs.gov/oei/reports/oei-05-12-00080.pdf. Accessed December 30, 2019.
34. White House O of M and B (OMB), White House O of M and B (OMB). Fiscal Year 2015 Budget of the U.S. Government. 2014. Available at: https://www.govinfo.gov/content/pkg/BUDGET-2015-BUD/pdf/BUDGET-2015-BUD.pdf. Accessed December 30, 2019.
35. Casey MM, Moscovice I, Holmes GM, et al. Minimum-distance requirements could harm high-performing critical-access hospitals and rural communities. Health Aff (Millwood) 2015;34(4):627–35.
36. Holmes GM, Pink GH, Friedman SA. The financial performance of rural hospitals and implications for elimination of the Critical Access Hospital program. J Rural Health 2013;29(2):140–9.
37. Williams D, Hadley J, Pettengill J. Profits, community role, and hospital closure: an urban and rural analysis. Med Care 1992;30(2):174–87.
38. Ciliberto F, Lindrooth RC. Exit from the hospital industry. Econ Inq 2007;45(1):71–81.
39. Lynn ML, Wertheim P. Key financial ratios can foretell hospital closures. Healthc Financ Manage 1993;47(11):66–70.
40. Ko M, Derose KP, Needleman J, et al. Whose social capital matters? The case of U.S. urban public hospital closures and conversions to private ownership. Soc Sci Med 2014;114:188–96.
41. Hsia RY, Kellermann AL, Shen Y-C. Factors associated with closures of emergency departments in the United States. JAMA 2011;305(19):1978–85.
42. Succi MJ, Lee SY, Alexander JA. Effects of market position and competition on rural hospital closures. Health Serv Res 1997;31(6):679–99.
43. McCue MJ, Clement JP. Assessing the characteristics of hospital bond defaults. Med Care 1996;34(11):1121–34.
44. Trussel JM, Patrick PA, DelliFraine J, et al. Rural hospital financial conditions: Evaluating Financial Distress in Rural Pennsylvania Hospitals. Available at: https://www.rural.palegislature.us/documents/reports/Rural_Hospital_Financial_2010.pdf. Accessed December 30, 2019.
45. Parker K, Horowits JM, Brown A, et al. Demographic and economic trends in urban, suburban and rural communities. Pew Res Center's Soc Demogr Trends Proj. May 2018. Available at: https://www.pewsocialtrends.org/2018/05/22/demographic-and-economic-trends-in-urban-suburban-and-rural-communities/. Accessed December 30, 2019.
46. TrendWatch: The Opportunities and Challenges for Rural Hospitals | AHA. American Hospital Association. Available at: https://www.aha.org/guidesreports/2011-04-18-trendwatch-opportunities-and-challenges-rural-hospitals. Accessed January 4, 2020.

47. Thomas SR, Holmes GM, Pink GH. 2012-14 Profitability of Urban and Rural Hospitals by Medicare Payment Classification. Available at: https://www.shepscenter.unc.edu/wp-content/uploads/dlm_uploads/2016/03/Profitability-of-Rural-Hospitals.pdf. Accessed December 30, 2019.
48. Jones CA, Parker TS, Ahearn M, et al. Health Status and Health Care Access of Farm and Rural Populations. Economic Information Bulletin No. 57. United States Department of Agriculture, Economic Research Service. 2009.
49. Middle Class Tax Relief and Job Creation Act of 2012 (2012 - H.R. 3630). GovTrack.us. Available at: https://www.govtrack.us/congress/bills/112/hr3630. Accessed January 4, 2020.
50. Summary of the Budget Control Act of 2011 | House Budget Committee Democrats. Available at: https://budget.house.gov/committee-report/summary-budget-control-act-2011. Accessed January 4, 2020.
51. Thompson K, Reiter K, Whitaker R, et al. Does ACA Insurance Coverage Expansion Improve the Financial Performance of Rural Hospitals? Available at: https://pdfs.semanticscholar.org/bde4/3f9a1a83d518bf284c1d5940a3772a47d7b4.pdf. Accessed January 4, 2020.
52. The Patient Protection and Affordable Care Act (PPACA), Pub. L. No. 111-148, 124 Stat. 119. 2010.
53. DSH fund cuts face difficult fight from hospitals. Modern Healthcare. 2019. Available at: https://www.modernhealthcare.com/politics-policy/dsh-fund-cuts-face-difficult-fight-hospitals. Accessed January 4, 2020.
54. Kaufman BG, Reiter KL, Pink GH, et al. Medicaid expansion affects rural and urban hospitals differently. Health Aff (Millwood) 2016;35(9):1665–72.
55. Pink GH, Freeman V, Randolph R, et al. Geographic Variation in the Profitability of Critical Access Hospitals. Available at: https://www.shepscenter.unc.edu/wp-content/uploads/2013/12/Geographic-Variation-in-the-Profitability-of-CAHs-Findings-Brief-Final_Sept-2013.pdf. Accessed December 30, 2019.
56. Pfuntner A, Wier LM, Stocks C. Most frequent procedures performed in U.S. hospitals, 2011: statistical brief #165. In: Healthcare cost and utilization project (HCUP) statistical briefs. Rockville (MD): Agency for Healthcare Research and Quality (US); 2006. Available at: http://www.ncbi.nlm.nih.gov/books/NBK174682/. Accessed November 24, 2017.
57. Gamm L, Hutchison L, Dabney B, et al. Rural healthy people 2010: a companion document to healthy people 2010, vol. 1. Tex AM Univ Syst Health Sci Cent Sch Rural Public Health Southwest Rural Health Res Cent; 2010. p. 275.
58. Chan L, Hart LG, Goodman DC. Geographic access to health care for rural Medicare beneficiaries. J Rural Health 2006;22(2):140–6.
59. Ellison EC, Pawlik TM, Way DP, et al. The impact of the aging population and incidence of cancer on future projections of general surgical workforce needs. Surgery 2018;163(3):553–9.
60. Ellison EC, Pawlik TM, Way DP, et al. Ten-year reassessment of the shortage of general surgeons: Increases in graduation numbers of general surgery residents are insufficient to meet the future demand for general surgeons. Surgery 2018;164(4):726–32.
61. Cohn SM, Price MA, Villarreal CL. Trauma and surgical critical care workforce in the united states: a severe surgeon shortage appears imminent. J Am Coll Surg 2009;209(4):446–52.e4.
62. Dall T, West T. The 2017 update: complexities of physician supply and demand: projections from 2015 to 2030. Washington, DC: IHS Markit; 2017. https://doi.org/10.13140/RG.2.2.16013.95209.

63. Williams TE, Satiani B, Ellison EC. A comparison of future recruitment needs in urban and rural hospitals: the rural imperative. Surgery 2011;150(4):617–25.
64. Aboagye JK, Kaiser HE, Hayanga AJ. Rural-urban differences in access to specialist providers of colorectal cancer care in the united states: a physician workforce issue. JAMA Surg 2014;149(6):537–43.
65. Bauder AR, Sarik JR, Butler PD, et al. Geographic variation in access to plastic surgeons. Ann Plast Surg 2016;76(2):238–43.
66. Polk HC, Bland KI, Ellison EC, et al. A proposal for enhancing the general surgical workforce and access to surgical care. Ann Surg 2012;255(4):611–7.
67. Diaz A, Merath K, Bagante F, et al. Surgical procedures in health professional shortage areas: impact of a surgical incentive payment plan. Surgery 2018; 164(2):189–94.
68. Shafi S, Aboutanos MB, Agarwal S, et al. Emergency general surgery: definition and estimated burden of disease. J Trauma Acute Care Surg 2013;74(4):1092–7.
69. Ingraham AM, Cohen ME, Raval MV, et al. Comparison of hospital performance in emergency versus elective general surgery operations at 198 hospitals. J Am Coll Surg 2011;212(1):20–8.e1.
70. Finks JF, Osborne NH, Birkmeyer JD. Trends in hospital volume and operative mortality for high-risk surgery. N Engl J Med 2011;364(22):2128–37.
71. Xu Z, Becerra AZ, Justiniano CF, et al. Is the distance worth it? patients with rectal cancer traveling to high-volume centers experience improved outcomes. Dis Colon Rectum 2017;60(12):1250–9.
72. Birkmeyer JD. Regionalization of high-risk surgery and implications for patient travel times. JAMA 2003;290(20):2703.
73. Diaz A, Schoenbrunner A, Cloyd J, et al. Geographic distribution of adult inpatient surgery capability in the USA. J Gastrointest Surg 2019. https://doi.org/10.1007/s11605-018-04078-9.
74. Ibrahim AM, Hughes TG, Thumma JR, et al. Association of hospital critical access status with surgical outcomes and expenditures among medicare beneficiaries. JAMA 2016;315(19):2095–103.
75. Gadzinski AJ, Dimick JB, Ye Z, et al. Utilization and outcomes of inpatient surgical care at critical access hospitals in the United States. JAMA Surg 2013;148(7): 589–96.
76. Finlayson SR, Birkmeyer JD, Tosteson AN, et al. Patient preferences for location of care: implications for regionalization. Med Care 1999;37(2):204–9.
77. Brooke BS, Goodney PP, Kraiss LW, et al. Readmission destination and risk of mortality after major surgery: an observational cohort study. Lancet 2015; 386(9996):884–95.
78. Reif SS, DesHarnais S, Bernard S. Community perceptions of the effects of rural hospital closure on access to care. J Rural Health 1999;15(2):202–9.
79. Critical Access Hospitals (CAHs) Introduction - Rural Health Information Hub. Available at: https://www.ruralhealthinfo.org/topics/critical-access-hospitals. Accessed December 30, 2019.
80. 340B Drug Pricing Program. 2017. Available at: https://www.hrsa.gov/opa/index.html. Accessed January 4, 2020.
81. Grassley CS. 1648 - 114th Congress (2015-2016): Rural Emergency Acute Care Hospital Act. 2015. Available at: https://www.congress.gov/bill/114th-congress/senate-bill/1648. Accessed December 30, 2019.
82. Graves S. H.R.2957 - 115th Congress (2017-2018): Save Rural Hospitals Act. 2017. Available at: https://www.congress.gov/bill/115th-congress/house-bill/2957. Accessed January 4, 2020.

83. Rural Emergency Acute Care Hospital Act (2017 - S. 1130). GovTrack.us. Available at: https://www.govtrack.us/congress/bills/115/s1130. Accessed January 4, 2020.
84. Save Rural Hospitals Act (2017 - H.R. 2957). GovTrack.us. Available at: https://www.govtrack.us/congress/bills/115/hr2957. Accessed January 4, 2020.
85. Federal Register Documents Currently on Public Inspection. Federal Register. Available at: https://www.federalregister.gov/public-inspection/current. Accessed January 4, 2020.

Initial and Ongoing Training of the Rural Surgeon

Gary L. Timmerman, MD[a,*], Thavam C. Thambi-Pillai, MD, MBA[a], Melissa K. Johnson, MD[b], John A. Weigelt, DVM, MD, MMA[c]

KEYWORDS

- Rural surgery • Training curriculum • Residency rotations • Surgical subspecialties
- General surgery • Frontier medicine

KEY POINTS

- Preparation for a practice in general surgery requires broad-based training with 10 prescribed core content areas. These goals are achieved through surgical rotations during residency.
- Active rural surgeons address gaps and deficiencies in residency training based on their current experiences. Additional skills are identified and included in current residency programs.
- Endoscopy has been demonstrated to realize the greatest percent increase in a rural surgeon's practice, providing evidence for greater exposure and training during residency.
- Many current residency programs have recognized the increasing shortage of rural general surgeons and therefore have restructured portions of their existing rotations to address the deficiencies.
- Continuing education and acquiring new technical skills remain a unique problem for the rural surgeon.

INTRODUCTION

In today's world of surgical specialization and subspecialization, defining a rural surgeon is a bit of a conundrum, and perhaps a disappointment owing to the departure from historical surgical training. Only a few decades ago, the definition of a general surgeon would truly encompass all the abilities, training and expectations of the rural surgeon. That individual would possess adequate knowledge and skills to manage most aspects of surgical diseases. This skill set extended into the fields of cardiothoracic, critical care, GI endoscopy, ENT, obstetrics/gynecology, orthopedics, plastic

[a] Department of Surgery, USD Sanford School of Medicine, Sanford Medical Center, Sioux Falls, SD 57105, USA; [b] Department of Surgery, USD Sanford School of Medicine, Royal C. Johnson Veterans Memorial Hospital, Sioux Falls, SD 57105, USA; [c] Department of Surgery, USD Sanford School of Medicine, Sioux Falls, SD 57105, USA
* Corresponding author.
E-mail address: Gary.Timmerman@Sanfordhealth.org

Surg Clin N Am 100 (2020) 849–859
https://doi.org/10.1016/j.suc.2020.06.004 surgical.theclinics.com
0039-6109/20/

surgery, trauma, urology and vascular. That individual has all but disappeared from our surgical profession.

The reasons behind this disappearance are multiple with external and internal changes to medicine. External pressures include expansion in technologic and pharmaceutical and medical advancements over the past 50 years, as well as greater patient expectations, improved life expectancy, and greater geographic mobility. Internal changes include development of subspecialty training in specific aspects of general surgery, as well as changes in resident training. The latter include the restriction on work hours as well as the expansion of surgical fellowships.

The changes in surgical education deserve special mention. The broad skill set a rural surgeon needs is more difficult to achieve in the current curriculum of residency training. Exposure to orthopedics, obstetrics and gynecology, and other surgical specialties is limited as training requirements have evolved away from a broad-based training paradigm. The ability to broadly prepare a future general surgeon for society's previous expectations within our current training curriculum is felt to be improbable and likely unobtainable. Another possible outcome of this shift in educational emphasis is decreased resident autonomy during the chief year with concerns that adequate preparation for independent surgical practice is elusive.

The Board of Governors and Young Fellows Association recently analyzed 2 on-line surveys regarding their members' opinion as to adequate training. More than 90% of young surgeons believed their training was adequate but in contrast, only 59% of older surgeons believed programs were providing adequate training.[1] Other factors identified as challenges for the rural surgeon included practice and lifestyle issues. Practice issues identified included call coverage, payer mix, reimbursement, malpractice risks, and employment models. Lifestyle issues focused on isolation from other surgeons, coverage expectations, and family contentment, as well as partner contentment. All of these factors contribute to the uncertainty for a well-trained general surgeon in a rural surgeon practice. Thus, it is no surprise that the number of general surgeons in rural areas has decreased by 26% over the past 25 years.[2] The number of graduating general surgery residents who enter the practice of general surgery is now around 200 or 20% of the graduating pool of surgeons. This number is not keeping up with the attrition rates of those retiring, in rural areas. This situation presents a manpower problem for surgical care across the United States, but especially in more rural states. A number of constructs have been proposed to address this shortage, starting with an examination of our surgical training programs.

Present American Board of Surgery Requirements for General/Rural Surgery Training

Preparation for general surgery still requires a relatively broad-based training with core content areas focusing on abdominal conditions, breast and endocrine disease, trauma and critical care, and surgical oncology. The American Board of Surgery (ABS) states that residency training in general surgery requires experience in 10 core content areas (**Box 1**). The ABS describes general surgery as a discipline that requires knowledge of and familiarity with a broad spectrum of diseases that may need surgical treatment. This knowledge requires attaining cognitive and skills training.

Cognitive training in these core content areas includes epidemiology, anatomy, physiology, pathology, and clinical presentation. Skills training includes technical proficiency when performing essential operations/procedures plus familiarity and technical proficiency with more uncommon and complex operations.[3]

The ABS, along with a consortium of groups dedicated to surgical education, developed the Surgical Council on Resident Education curriculum to address the vast array

Box 1
Core content areas of general surgery defined by the ABS, February 2017

Alimentary tract (including bariatric surgery)

Abdomen and its contents

Breast, skin, and soft tissue

Endocrine system

Solid organ transplantation

Pediatric surgery

Surgical critical care

Surgical oncology (including head and neck surgery)

Trauma, burns, and emergency surgery

Vascular surgery

Courtesy of Accreditation Council for Graduate Medical Education (ACGME), Chicago, IL.

of diseases/conditions and procedures/operations that are included in these 10 core content areas.[4] This curriculum attempts to impart cognitive knowledge and operative skills with surgical judgment. Measurement of cognitive knowledge occurs by various tests and oral presentations. Objective measures of performance in the operating room are based on a standardized assessment of key technical steps and surgical decisions in index procedures. Whether simulation approaches will make this task easier remains to be seen. As our medical community has become more complex, training is now necessary in patient safety, quality assessment, professionalism, and communication skills. The 6 Accreditation Council for Graduate Medical Education competencies emphasize these additional training goals:

1. Patient care
2. Medical knowledge
3. System-based practice
4. Practice-based learning and improvement
5. Professionalism
6. Interpersonal and communications skills[5]

This curriculum also established minimal numbers of procedures for a finishing general surgery resident (**Table 1**). General surgery residents must report a minimum of 850 operative cases during training and at least 200 during the chief residency year. Up to 25 cases as teaching assistant may count toward the total 850 cases. The ABS and Residency Review Committee for Surgery established the number of cases for each category to qualify for ABS certification. How well these procedures align with the needs of a general/rural surgeon is questionable.[6]

ALTERNATIVE OPTIONS FOR RURAL SURGERY TRAINING

General surgery training implies the trainee is exposed to and needs to assimilate this broad-based surgical education. However, is the current training process adequate for the patient care issues a rural general surgeon encounters? The rural general surgeon needs a broad-based experience in general surgery, but they also require experience in conditions and procedures outside the ABS description of general surgery.

Table 1
Defined category minimum numbers for general surgery residents and credit role review committee for surgery

Category	Minimum
Skin, soft tissue	25
Breast	40
Mastectomy	5
Axilla	5
Head and neck	25
Alimentary tract	180
Esophagus	5
Stomach	15
Small intestine	25
Large intestine	40
Appendix	40
Anorectal	20
Abdominal	250
Biliary	85
Hernia	85
Liver	5
Pancreas	5
Vascular	50
Access	10
Anastomosis, repair or endarterectomy	10
Endocrine	15
Thyroid or parathyroid	10
Operative trauma	10
Nonoperative trauma	40
Resuscitations as team leader	10
Thoracic surgery	20
Thoracotomy	5
Pediatric surgery	20
Plastic surgery	10
Surgical critical care	40
Laparoscopic basic	100
Endoscopy	85
Upper endoscopy	35
Colonoscopy	50
Laparoscopic complex	75
Total major cases	850
Chief year major cases	200
Teaching assistant cases	25

Courtesy of Accreditation Council for Graduate Medical Education (ACGME), Chicago, IL.

Conditions and skills in the fields of obstetrics, orthopedics, plastic surgery, urology, and otolaryngoscopy are needed.[7] Basic training in trauma/critical care is beneficial. Yet, the current general surgery training offers little opportunity for achieving information regarding basic principles of recognizing problems within these areas.

Curriculum Based on the Rural Surgeon's Needs Assessment

A needs assessment may help to define a training paradigm for a rural general surgeon and identify gaps in their current experience. Rural surgeons were solicited for their opinions as to the skill set required to embark on a rural surgery career. This survey included more than 230 practicing rural surgeons, of whom more than 60% had been in practice for more than 20 years. The most valuable skills identified were endoscopy, advanced laparoscopy, and basic nongeneral surgery subspecialty procedures. Respondents also believed a rural surgery experience during residency was highly valuable (82%). Finally, there was overwhelming support for training programs that offered broad general surgery experience, high case volumes, and no or few fellows competing in the subspecialties.[8]

Curriculum Based on Case Log Evaluations

Another way to explore the practice needs of a rural general surgeon is to study the case logs of surgeons with established practices in rural America. Sticca and colleagues[7] collated the surgical procedures performed by all surgeons in North Dakota and South Dakota in 2006. Surgeons were classified as rural or urban. Rural surgeons performed an average of 1071 procedures, including endoscopy (39%), general surgery (26%), minor surgery (18%), and surgical subspecialty cases (12%). Cholecystectomy (6.3%), hernia repair (6.2%), breast surgery (4.9%), and appendectomy (2.2%) were the major procedures performed. A subanalysis of the surgical subspecialty procedures made up 12.3% and revealed that the most frequent of these were vascular (37%), obstetrics/gynecology (19%), orthopedics (15%), cardiothoracic (11%), urology (9%), and otolaryngology (4%).[7]

In 2019, a similar upper Midwest patient population was evaluated for current trends in surgical procedures performed in a rural setting (population <50,000). Six Minnesota and South Dakota rural hospitals were included. The operative case volumes and subspecialty procedures were examined at these 6 rural communities from January 2013 through August 2018. A total of 38,958 procedures were performed at those locations by 58 general surgeons.

Each facility performed an average of 1180 cases per year. The data provided a snapshot of surgical practice. Endoscopic procedures accounted for 62% of surgeon activity, which was increased by more than 20% from the 2006 study. Cholecystectomy (6.3%), herniorraphy (6.3%), and appendectomy (3.7%) were the most common major procedures. When combined with endoscopy, these 4 interventions comprised nearly 80% of today's rural surgeon's caseload.[9] Some interesting decreases declines in activity were also noted. Colorectal and breast surgeries comprised only 2.3% and 1.8% of cases, respectively, compared with 6.0% and 4.9% in 2006 and 5.6% and 3.1% from another 2014 rural case analysis.[10]

Subspecialty procedures are also declining in the rural setting. They decreased from 12.3% in 2006 to less than 5% in 2019. Decreases were also noted in obstetrics/gynecology, urology, and vascular procedures (**Table 2**).

This trend is disturbing because it seems that rural surgery with subspecialty surgical care is withering in smaller communities in the United States. The cause is not entirely clear. One explanation is that we are not preparing current trainees for a practice focused for these communities. Frequently, these rural locations may

Table 2
Subspecialty rates from 3 comparisons (case analysis)

Subspecialty	2006 (% Cases)	2014 (% Cases)	2019 (% Cases)
Obstetrics/gynecology	2.3	0.7	0.4
Urology	1.1	0.5	0.2
Vascular	4.6	3.7	2.5

have only 1 obstetrics/gynecology or perhaps 1 orthopedic surgeon for which considerations for call coverage or backup dictates the rural surgeon's operative privileges. Many smaller communities now offer daytime specialty outreach clinics, again with the expectation that night and week-end call coverage will be provided by the rural surgeon for these specialties. For this reason, many rural-minded residency programs offer additional opportunities in those specific specialties during or immediately after residency to prepare the graduating chief resident for their upcoming employment. Another explanation is that our health care systems are forcing patients to make choices about where they seek their health care. Either places a burden on patients and health care providers. How to provide an appropriate level of safe broad-based surgical care to smaller US communities is the real question. Solutions are not easy to identify, but a logical place to start is with the training of future surgeons.

Curriculum Based on Alternative Rural Surgery Residency Training Models

As medical schools and training programs recognized the shortage of rural general surgeons, they restructured part of their training programs attempting to address this shortage. Change for medical students is often a rotation in a smaller community with a practicing surgeon to entice and show the student the benefits of a rural practice. For residents, a similar exposure helps them to define what they will experience in a rural practice and the skill set necessary to be successful and enjoy the experience. Another strategy is "loan forgiveness" plans in exchange for a prescribed period of time practicing in rural communities. Recently, the American College of Surgeons proposed 3 opportunities to address this growing crisis:

1. "Fix-the-five";
2. Create new surgical residencies with primary focus in rural surgery; and
3. Create "Transitions to Practice" fellowships (Mastery in General Surgery Programs).[11]

The fix-the-five means adding rural surgery opportunities as electives available to any residents interested in rural surgery during the traditional 5 to 7 years of surgical training. Numerous institutions located in both rural and urban regions have created 1- to 3-month AWAY rural surgery rotations at small or rural communities with a practicing surgeon. Recently, this program was extended to developing countries with either rural and/or global surgical health care intentions. This rotation is often part of the general curriculum for all residents. These rotations tend to occur during the second to fourth years of surgical residency.

Other institutions have created a dedicated rural surgery track, where up to 9 months of training, including rural surgery rotations and surgical subspecialty training, are provided to interested residents again during their second through fourth years. This is a specific program and can be available through the National Residency Matching Program as a distinct and separate entity.[12] Finally, in an attempt to fix-the-five, the Oregon Health Sciences University and University of Utah created an immersion approach, in which interested residents may spend an entire year in a rural community in lieu of a usual year of research during the middle years of their residency. These experiences also offer subspecialty training usually free of competing specialty residents for greater exposure and hands-on opportunity.[13,14]

General surgery programs that are just starting provide another opportunity to train rural general surgeons. New programs must meet all the Accreditation Council for Graduate Medical Education requirements for general surgery, but they also recognize and meet the educational and specific training needs of a rural surgeon. This goal is often easy to accomplish because these programs are commonly located in more rural areas of our country. Another unique characteristic is the lack of subspecialty residents allowing the general surgery residents to gain experience in many different specialties. Such programs offer higher volumes of endoscopy and ambulatory surgical exposure, commensurate with the typical rural surgeon's case log.

Finally, many institutions have created general surgery "fellowship" opportunities. These fellowships are identified as Transitions to Practice or Mastery in General Surgery Programs. Transitions to Practice allow a graduated general surgery resident to spend additional time (6 months to 2 years) for greater focused surgical experiences, such as endoscopy, subspecialty exposure, or greater independent surgical experiences. This fellowship is believed to broaden competence and develop the confidence necessary to practice in rural regions or communities.[15]

Irrespective of the curriculum training model, the management and care of the trauma patient remains absolutely critical for the rural surgeon, who may serve as the first contact in designated or nondesignated trauma centers. Rural surgeons serve as community leaders to coordinate local trauma care. They provide the necessary procedures and techniques to accomplish resuscitation and stabilization, triage patients for transfer to trauma centers, and provide definitive care when appropriate.[16]

Not all curricula are met with obvious success in training or promoting rural surgery opportunities. Other countries from around the world also struggle with enrollment and training surgeons for practice as rural surgeons. One such country is Australia, where a significant proportion of citizens (31%) live in nonmetropolitan locations. In 2009, only 22% of general surgeons were practicing in rural or remote areas. Our colleagues from the Royal Australasian College of Surgeons developed a Rural Surgical Training Program with the objective of supporting recruitment and offering specialized training to residents for rural surgical practice. This program ran from 1996 to 2007 and was evaluated thereafter. Unfortunately, the project was felt not to adequately prepare trainees for rural surgery, nor did it result in those same individuals practicing in rural Australia (only 23%). The Rural Surgical Training Program did little to influence the trainee's career choices or retain the individuals in rural practice. Although the Rural Surgical Training Program as initially conceived was deemed a failure, insight was gained that targeting trainees upon entering residency may be too late to sway the trainees future practice intentions.[17]

In an attempt to expose future physicians to rural practice before residency selection, including primary care and rural surgery, some medical schools have purposely created an immersion rural clinical training experience for several selected MS-3 students. In 1971, the University of Minnesota created the Rural Physician Associate Program to address their shortage of primary care in that state. A 9-month MS-3 year community based educational experience was created that exposed the students to live and train in rural communities in Minnesota and western Wisconsin. Students interested in family medicine or primary care interview and between 19 to 46 students per year are selected, 1 student to each community with board-certified medical physician instructors. This program now boast more than 1500 alumni with 66% practicing in Minnesota, 40% in rural communities, and 75% practicing primary care.[18,19]

Similarly, the University of South Dakota Sanford School of Medicine created the FARM (Frontier and Rural Medicine) track which places 9 Pillar II (MS-3) students in 7 rural locations where students participate in the full spectrum of rural medical and surgical care.

Since 2014, 34 students have completed the program with 40% going on to enter family medicine residencies and 20% have entered the primary care fields of internal medicine, pediatrics, or obstetrics/gynecology.[20] Although promising, it is too early to comment if this project will lead to a successful transition to an actual rural practice.

Finally, many rural and general surgeons contribute their time and efforts performing "missionary" or global clinical surgery to underserved or developing world nations, where the surgeon represents the only standard of care for that community or locale. Several US programs have enlisted in global clinical surgical education programs with the goal of expanding access and quality surgical health care to low-income and underserved countries. One such program is the Alliance for Global Clinical Training (consisting of surgical educators and residents from several programs affiliated with the Pacific Coast Surgical Association) and Muhimbili University of Health and Allied Sciences/Muhimbili National Hospital in Salaam, Tanzania. This consortium developed collaborative relationships between high-income country faculty surgeons and residents with those low-income countries to offer 1-month rotations with several unique objectives including (1) exposure to surgical practice in a resource-constrained environment, (2) exposure to the challenges of cross-cultural clinical practice, (3) exposure to acute surgical abdomens and advanced malignancy not routinely encountered in Western practice, and (4) exposure to open surgery and hand-sewn intestinal anastomoses now infrequently experienced in Western surgery residency programs. Given the advanced nature of surgical care, course leaders felt this rotation was best for residents in their third year and beyond.[21] Although the expectations of the endeavor are met, there seems to be greater (and expected) benefit to the low-income countries facility and patient population than preparing high-income country surgeons for global or rural surgical careers.

Many investigators have likened global surgical care and its training to rural surgical training given their similar clinical exposure, isolationism, and broad surgical training requirements. Certainly, individuals looking for a career in either clinical practice seek out programs with similar training opportunities.

Maintaining Competence and Life-Long Learning for Rural Surgeons

Another issue is maintaining competence and life-long learning for a rural surgeon. Rural surgeons truly have unique and challenging learning barriers different from the continuous professional development courses available to other surgeons. All surgeons are required to maintain professional certification in their specialty. General surgeons most commonly do this by maintaining board certification from the ABS. This method aims at ensuring the surgeon is up to date on their medical knowledge. Many barriers exist for the rural general surgeon in accomplishing this recertification.

Staying current in medicine is a challenge for all surgeons, especially with the rapid changes in today's knowledge base. Spending time away from their practice is difficult for rural surgeons to attend continuing medical education courses. This time away means a lack of surgical backup for their community and the loss of income. Thoughtful and deliberate modifications to traditional educational courses have been created by teams of large academic and rural surgeons along with individuals with expertise in adult education. Much of this learning can now be accessed electronically without the need for surgeons to leave their community. This change will certainly help rural general surgeons to maintain their medical knowledge base.

Advances in technology are another challenge. Laparoscopic surgery dramatically changed the approach to abdominal surgery and has contributed significantly to patient expectations and the quality of care. Most recently, robotic surgery has become another technical approach that is being used as a marketing and recruitment tool for hospitals and medical staffs.

Traditionally, nearly all surgeons travel to various urban or other locations to attend discipline-specific updates to acquire or maintain new surgical education or technical skills within their chosen field of practice. These events are typically sponsored by the American College of Surgeons, other surgical specialty societies, or even medical device industries across the United States or abroad. Recently, skills courses sponsored through the Nora Institute Advanced Skills Course for Rural Surgeons were developed through a needs assessment from rural surgeons for content or training. These courses may either refresh older but infrequently used skills or train new techniques or technical offerings. The courses often take to the road, bringing the surgical update or education opportunity directly to the rural surgeon or to nearby locations.[22] Examples of learning modules include endoscopic skills such as foreign body removal, advanced polypectomy techniques, stricture dilation, and stent placement. Other learning modules encompass emergency gynecology, emergency urology, breast ultrasound examination, ultrasound examination for central line placement, advanced plastic surgery repairs, and laparoscopic common bile duct explorations.[23,24]

Surgical telementoring, consisting of an expert surgeon guiding either a less experienced surgeon through an advanced case or teaching a new technique to a rural surgeon from a remote location, is an evolving technology with potential educational benefits. Telemedicine has experienced a steady implementation for emergency medicine, medical specialty care, cardiology, and rural trauma care where no specialist or surgeon is on staff. One hundred fifty-nine surgeons, 82% of whom practice in communities of less than 50,000 people, recently completed a survey. Nearly 80% felt telementoring would be useful to their practice and most believed beneficial to their hospital. When surgeons were queried about the single most useful application of surgical telementoring, 46.5% picked learning new techniques or skill sets and 39% chose intraoperative assistance with unexpected findings. When asked to select applications they would be willing to use telementoring from a list of other possible uses, surgeons most frequently selected consultation for unexpected findings, trauma consultation, and laparoscopic colectomy. This technology is felt by many to be on the verge of widespread use.[25]

SUMMARY

The initial and ongoing training of the rural surgeon remains an enigma. There is neither a solid or confirmed curriculum for the training of an individual with the necessary knowledge or skill set to successfully master a rural surgical practice. Multiple curricula and training programs are being tried but no long term results exist to validate a best approach.

It is recognized that general surgery residency requires attaining an increasing amount of surgical knowledge and skill sets. The curriculum is crowded and imparting the core knowledge and skills to our residents is a challenge. A variety of modifications to current training curriculums are under careful evaluation and scrutiny. The goal is to sculpt a rural surgical residency experience within general surgery residencies allowing some trainees to finish with knowledge and skills better suited for a current rural surgical practice. Unfortunately, the optimal modifications within our residency programs to achieve this goal remains elusive.

DISCLOSURE

The authors have nothing to disclose.

REFERENCES

1. Napolitano L, Paramo J, Savarise M, et al. Are General Surgery Residents Ready to Practice? A Survey of the American College of Surgeons Board of Governors and Young Fellows Association. J Am Coll Surg 2014;218(5):1063–72.
2. Fischer JE. How to rescue general surgery (editorial opinion). Am J Surg 2012; 204:541–2.
3. Available at: https://www.absurgery.org/default.jsp?certgsqe_essentials Last. Accessed January 07, 2020.
4. Available at: https://www.absurgery.org/xfer/curriculumoutline2018-19.pdf Last. Accessed January 07, 2020.
5. Available at: https://www.acgme.org/Portals/0/PFAssets/ProgramRequirements/440_GeneralSurgery_2019_TCC.pdf?ver=2019-05-03-123758-307 Last. Accessed January 07, 2020.
6. Available at: https://www.acgme.org/Portals/0/DefinedCategoryMinimumNumbersforGeneralSurgeryResidentsandCreditRole.pdf Last. Accessed January 07, 2020.
7. Sticca RP, Mullin BC, Harris JD, et al. Surgical specialty procedures in rural surgery practices: implications for rural surgery training. Am J Surg 2012;204(6): 1007–12.
8. Deal SB, Cook MR, Hughes D, et al. Training for a Career in Rural and Nonmetropolitan Surgery-A Practical Needs Assessment. J Surg Educ 2018;75(6): e229–33.
9. Stinson W, Timmerman G, Bjordahl P, et al. Current trends in surgical procedures performed in rural general surgery practice. Accepted for publication, The American Surgeon; 2020.
10. Perl VU, Diggs B, Ham B, et al. Does surgery residency prepare residents to work at critical access hospitals? Am J Surg 2015;209(5):828–32.
11. Deveney K, Jarman B, Sticca R. Responding to the need for rural general surgery training sites: a how-to. Bull Am Coll Surg 2015;100(4):47–50.
12. Mercier PJ, Skube SJ, Leonard SL, et al. Creating a Rural Surgery Track and a Review of Rural Surgery Training Programs. J Surg Educ 2019;76(2):459–68.
13. Hunter JG, Deveney KE. Training the rural surgeon: a proposal. Bull Am Coll Surg 2003;88(5):13–7.
14. Deveney K, Deatherage M, Oehling D, et al. Association between dedicated rural training year and the likelihood of becoming a general surgeon in a small town. JAMA Surg 2013;148(9):817–21.
15. Borgstrom DC. Rural surgical practice requires new training model, offers great opportunities. Bull Am Coll Surg 2013;98(7):55–6.
16. Cogbill TH, Cofer JB, Jarman GT. Contemporary issues in rural surgery. Curr Probl Surg 2012 May;49(5):263–318.
17. Chong A, Kiroff G. Preparing surgeons for rural Australia: the RACS Rural Surgical Training Program. ANZ J Surg 2015;85(3):108–12.
18. Zink T, Center B, Finstad D, et al. Efforts to graduate more primary care physicians and physicians who will practice in rural areas: examining outcomes from

the University of Minnesota-Duluth and the rural physician associate program. Acad Med 2010;85(5):599–604.
19. Available at: https://med.umn.edu/md-students/individualized-pathways/rural-physician-associate-program-rpap. Accessed January 07, 2020.
20. Anderson S. Frontier and Rural Medicine (FARM) Program. S D Med 2019;72(7):292–3.
21. Graf J, Cook M, Schecter S, et al. Coalition for Global Clinical Surgical Education: The Alliance for Global Clinical Training. J Surg Educ 2018;75(3):688–96.
22. Available at: http://bulletin.facs.org/2016/04/skills-course-helps-rural-surgeons-stay-current/. Accessed January 07, 2020.
23. Halverson AL, DaRosa DA, Borgstrom DC, et al. Evaluation of a blended learning surgical skills course for rural surgeons. Am J Surg 2014;208(1):136–42.
24. Halverson AL, Hughes TG, Borgstrom DC, et al. What surgical skills rural surgeons need to master. J Am Coll Surg 2013;217(5):919–23.
25. Glenn IC, Bruns NE, Hayek D, et al. Rural surgeons would embrace surgical telementoring for help with difficult cases and acquisition of new skills. Surg Endosc 2017;31(3):1264–8.

Scope of Practice of the Rural Surgeon

Mary Oline Aaland, MD*

KEYWORDS

• Strong surgical foundation • Flexibility • Community involvement

KEY POINTS

- Practicing in a rural community requires a strong foundation in all aspects of surgical care—preoperative, operative, and postoperative.
- The rural surgeon must be flexible and creative to develop a surgical program specific to the needs of the community.
- Partnering with the community leaders is key to developing a rewarding rural surgical practice.

INTRODUCTION

The purpose of this section of the Surgical Clinics is to describe the scope of practice of the rural surgeon. Literature is sparse because rural surgeons are often not in the habit of publishing papers. Therefore, there are 3 segments to this discussion: (1) a review of the current published literature for the last decade; (2) a brief description of several rural practices across the United States; and (3) a look to the future with the changes in the overall delivery of surgical care and the possible benefit to rural surgeons.

Review of the Current (2010–2019) Published Literature

One of the few comprehensive reviews of case volume development of a rural surgery network was published from Wisconsin in 2017.[1] Cogbill and his colleagues at the Gunderson Health System have developed a sustainable rural surgery model with partnerships with Critical Assess Hospitals (CAH) within a 3 state rural area-southwestern Wisconsin, southeastern Minnesota, and northeastern Iowa. That program has been in existence for 38 years. In that report, they summarized the operative case mix for the surgeons that practice at the surrounding CAHs for 2016 (**Table 1**). The case mix was 63.8% endoscopy, 26.7% general surgery, and 6.1% obstetrics and gynecology. This change was significant from their published data from 20 years

Department of Surgery, University of North Dakota, Grand Forks, ND, USA
* 1103 Broadway N, Fargo, ND 58102.
E-mail address: Mary.aaland@und.edu

Surg Clin N Am 100 (2020) 861–868
https://doi.org/10.1016/j.suc.2020.06.002
0039-6109/20/

Table 1
Operative case mix for current Gundersen Health System rural general surgeons

Procedure	Proportion of Operative Case Mix, %
Colonoscopy	52.6
Esophagogastroduodenoscopy	11.2
Excisions and wound care	8.2
Hernias	5.9
Cesarean section	3.9
Cholecystectomy	3.6
Appendectomy	3.3
Gynecology	2.2
Colectomy	1.2
Vasectomy	1.2
Vascular access	1
Anorectal	0.9
Breast	0.7
Miscellaneous	4.1
Total	100

From Cogbill TH, Bintz M. Rural General Surgery: A 38-Year Experience with a Regional Network Established by an Integrated Health System in the Midwestern United States. Journal of the American College of Surgeons. 2017;225(1):115-123; with permission.

earlier, where their rural surgeons performed 31% general surgery, 28% endoscopy, 26% obstetrics and gynecology, and 15% surgical subspecialty cases.[2] They did not have a clear reason why there was such a change during the last 2 decades.

Although published in 2010, the scope of practice outlined by Harris and colleagues[3] from North Dakota and South Dakota, the data were similar to the findings of Cogbill from Wisconsin. The case mix in that study was 40% endoscopy, 26% general surgery, 18% minor surgery, and 12% surgical specialty.

The Department of Surgery and Division of Trauma, Critical Care & Acute Surgery from Oregon Health & Science University in Portland Oregon compared operations performed at CAH verses the case logs of the university-based surgical residents for 2013 to 2014 in an attempt to determine if their training program was adequately preparing surgical residents to enter a rural practice.[4] Data were extracted from the Oregon Association of Hospital and Health Systems database for 2012 to 2013 using National Provider Identification to determine what surgical procedures were being performed at the CAHs. This methodology allowed them to compare the procedures performed by the senior surgical residents with the general surgeons that performed surgeries at the CAHs in Oregon (**Table 2**).

The top 10 procedures for the general surgeons from that study are listed below.

1. Endoscopy, 56.1%
2. Hernia, 8.8%
3. Cholecystectomy/common bile duct, 6.4%
4. Skin/soft tissue, 5.4%
5. Small/large bowel, 4.0%
6. Breast, 3.1%
7. Appendix, 2.4%

Table 2
Procedures excluding endoscopy

	Surgery Residents, Nonendoscopy (%)	General Surgeons, Nonendoscopy (%)	*P* Value
General surgery procedures			
Appendix	6.1	5.6	.024
Breast	5.1	7	<.001
Cholecystectomy/ common bile duct	9.9	14.6	<.001
Endocrine	2.2	0.5	<.001
Endoscopy	–	–	
Esophagus/stomach	3.9	2.3	<.001
Hernia	11.7	20	<.001
Liver/pancreas	2.5	0.7	<.001
Other abdominal	7.5	4.6	<.001
Rectal/anal	1.1	3.6	<.001
Skin/soft tissue	7.8	12.6	<.001
Small/large bowel	13.6	9.2	<.001
Spleen/lymph	3.1	2.3	<.001
Trachea	1.1	0	<.001
Surgery specialty procedures			
Cardiothoracic	5.6	1.9	<.001
Neurosurgery	0.2	0.8	<.001
Obstetrics and gynecology	0.5	1.5	<.001
Ophthalmology	0	0.1	0.004
Orthopedics	4.6	2.8	<.001
Otolaryngology	0.5	0.3	.001
Urology	0.8	1.2	<.001
Vascular	12.1	8.4	<.001
Total	99.9	100	

From Undurraga Perl V, Diggs B, Ham B, Schreiber M. Does surgery residency prepare residents to work at critical access hospitals? American Journal Of Surgery. 2015;209(5):828-832; with permission.

8. Other abdominal, 2.0%
9. Rectal/anal, 1.6%
10. Esophagus/stomach, 1.0%

In comparing the senior surgical resident's operative experience with that of the CAH surgeons, the CAH surgeons performed a higher proportion for endoscopies than the surgical residents (56.1% vs 9.1%). However, the CAH rural surgeons did a higher percentage of general surgery (92.4% vs 77.8%). This study included **Table 3**, which lists the procedures excluding endoscopy for the years noted. The conclusion of that analysis after reviewing the scope of practice of the surgeons that practiced at CAHs was that surgical residents that are interested in practicing in rural surgery would benefit from increased case load in areas such as endoscopy, hernia, breast, and cholecystectomy/common bile duct procedures during their training.

Table 3
Procedures performed by surgery residents graduating in 2013 and 2014 and general surgeons at Critical Access Hospitals (2012–2013)

	Surgery Residents, All Procedures (%)	General Surgeons, All Procedures (%)	*P* Value
General surgery procedures			
Appendix	1779 (5.6)	839 (2.4)	<.001
Breast	1485 (4.6)	1048 (3.1)	<.001
Cholecystectomy/ common bile duct	2872 (9.0)	2190 (6.4)	<.001
Endocrine	638 (2.0)	73 (.2)	<.001
Endoscopy	2920 (9.1)	19,225 (56.1)	<.001
Esophagus/stomach	1144 (3.6)	343 (1.0)	<.001
Hernia	3400 (10.6)	3006 (8.8)	<.001
Liver/pancreas	714 (2.2)	110 (.3)	<.001
Other abdominal	2171 (6.8)	693 (2.0)	<.001
Rectal/anal	330 (1.0)	539 (1.6)	<.001
Skin/soft tissue	2275 (7.1)	1897 (5.5)	<.001
Small/large bowel	3953 (12.4)	1381 (4.0)	<.001
Spleen/lymph	904 (2.8)	345 (1.0)	<.001
Trachea	329 (1.0)	2 (.0)	<.001
Surgery specialty procedures			
Cardiothoracic	1628 (5.1)	289 (.8)	<.001
Neurosurgery	48 (.2)	124 (.4)	<.001
Obstetrics and gynecology	142 (.4)	227 (.7)	<.001
Ophthalmology	7 (.0)	13 (.0)	<.001
Orthopedics	1335 (4.2)	427 (1.2)	<.001
Otolaryngology	141 (.4)	41 (.1)	<.001
Urology	240 (.8)	179 (.5)	<.001
Vascular	3522 (11.0)	1255 (3.7)	<.001
Total	31,977 (99.9)	34,246 (99.8)	

From Undurraga Perl V, Diggs B, Ham B, Schreiber M. Does surgery residency prepare residents to work at critical access hospitals? American Journal Of Surgery. 2015;209(5):828-832; with permission.

Not all rural hospitals are CAHs, such as the Mary Lanning Memorial Hospital in Hastings, Nebraska. That rural community hospital had 161 beds and 3 general surgeons when they published their surgical experience.[5] Each surgeon performed approximately 561 procedures per year. The 10 most commonly performed procedures between 2008 and 2010 were:

1. Colonoscopy and esophagogastroduodenoscopy
2. Laparoscopic and open cholecystectomy
3. Insertion of venous access port
4. Hernia repair
5. Laparoscopic appendectomy
6. Exploratory laparotomy and bowel resection
7. Debridement of the lower extremity

8. Breast lumpectomy
9. Mastectomy
10. Laparoscopic colon resection

Rural Surgical Practices Across America

As stated in the beginning of this article, publications from the last 10 years are sparse on what is the scope of practice in rural America, although more than 60 million Americans live in a rural setting. The next segment of this section of the Scope of Practice of the Rural Surgeons briefly discusses several rural surgical practices across America.

There are many more success stories of small community-based hospitals with strong general surgical presence across the United States that have untold stories and unshared data. Without these rural surgeons and nonacademic surgical practices, patient care would be compromised. The scope of practice in these communities is as varied as the communities that are served.

J. David Richardson, MD, FACS, professor of surgery at University of Louisville School of Medicines, Kentucky, and former President of the American College of Surgeons (ACS) has long been a champion of the rural surgeon. In an interview published in the 2015 ACS October Bulletin, he stated, "I can remember when I had a perforated appendix at age 10 and had a two-and-a-half hour ride to Lexington (KY) in a pickup truck in the pre-interstate highway days." He went on to say, "I always remembered how scared I was and how uncomfortable it was." In his hometown of Morehead, Kentucky, there was no hospital until he was 18 years of age. As a second-year surgical resident, he spent 3 months with the local surgeon and gained a respect for the surgical care provided. That rural community has continued to grow. He concluded that, "There is outstanding surgical care. We've got specialty surgeons now. We've got four general surgeons, and they do a great job."[6]

Jamestown, North Dakota, has a CAH that is located 100 miles from any large city. The community itself has had a relatively stable population of roughly 15,000 people. The hospital was built 1929 and has remained open since then. In 2008, a completely new campus was built. To date, there are 3 general surgeons, 2 urologists, 2 orthopedic surgeons, and 1 ENT.

Hopedale, Illinois, with a population of less than 1000, has a CAH that is a true success story of what talented surgeons can develop in a small community. General, vascular, and orthopedic surgeries are provided, as well as extensive medical services.

Perhaps a window into these practices can be implied by the on-line survey of practicing rural surgeons that subscribe to the ACS Rural Surgery listserv recently published by Deal and colleagues.[7] This survey was done to attempt to perform a practical needs assessment. The majority of the 237 rural surgeons that responded had more than 20 years of experience and were from 49 states. **Table 4** summarizes the procedural training for subspecialty skills that the responding rural surgeons recommended. This list goes well beyond endoscopy to include urology, orthopedics, ENT, obstetrics, and plastics. These nontraditional procedures that would nominally be considered specialist only in urban climes provide a window into the scope of practice of our rural surgical colleagues.

A Look to the Future with the Changes that Are Occurring in Surgical Care and How It Could Benefit the Rural Surgeon

With the limited documentation of the scope of practice of the rural surgeon, clearer impressions of the types of practices in the nonmetropolitan centers has been defined by the work of Cook and colleagues.[8] Again, using the ACS rural listserv,

Table 4
Recommended procedural training for subspecialty skills based on free-response textual analysis

Specialty	Procedure
Obstetrics and gynecology	Cesarean section Emergent hysterectomy Tubal ligation Dilation and curettage
Urology	Ureteral stent placement Suprapubic catheter placement Vasectomy Bladder suspension Cystoscopy
Gastroenterology	Colonoscopy Upper endoscopy Bleeding control techniques and biopsy Stenting Endoscopic retrograde cholangiopancreatography
Breast	Oncoplastic techniques Stereotactic breast biopsy Ultrasound examination
Orthopedics	Carpal tunnel release Ganglion cyst management Traumatic amputation Dislocation management Common fracture management
ENT	Tonsillectomy
Plastics	Simple rotational flap Complex laceration repair

From Deal SB, Cook MR, Hughes D, et al. Training for a Career in Rural and Nonmetropolitan Surgery—A Practical Needs Assessment. Journal of Surgical Education. 2018;75(6):e229-e233; with permission.

a survey was sent out to the members, of which 237 responded to the 15-item survey. Seventy-two percent of the respondents practiced in communities with a population of less than 50,000 and 85% had been in practice for more than 10 years. That analysis stated "Rural surgery is practiced in communities of less than 50,000; and large nonmetropolitan practices exist in nonurban communities of greater than 100,000. There is a continuum of practices between these sizes, and traditional, dichotomous definitions of rural versus urban practices may no longer adequately describe the diversity of nonmetropolitan general surgery being practiced in the United States." In this group of surveyed surgeons, 51% agreed that there is benefit to additional subspecialty training for a surgical resident interested in a rural practice. Again, this finding could be reflective of what cases are currently being done in the smaller communities. In very small communities, available hospital resources often are the limiting factor for expanding the scope of practice, but this study in the larger "rural" hospitals it seems that the scope of practice could be further expanded by subspecialization.

In the CAH, maintaining operating room staff 24/7 is not logistically possible, but this is not the end of the world in terms of broad-based surgical work because there has been a fundamental shift in inpatient/outpatient surgery. In the United Stated today, ambulatory surgery has exploded. In 1994, 57% of surgeries done in community hospitals were done in the ambulatory surgery centers. In 2014, this number had increased to 66%.[9] In that document, the top 25 most common ambulatory invasive, therapeutic surgeries performed in the community hospitals included 8 that would be considered in the general surgeon's scope of practice (biliary, hernias, tonsillectomy, breast, catheter placements, appendectomy, lymph node, and hysterectomies). With the advent of laparoscopic colectomy being a short stay procedure, these procedures increasingly require fewer hospital resources.

With the increasing emphasis on cost and value of care, Imran and colleagues[10] demonstrated that ambulatory surgery center outpatient procedures are more efficient than those performed in the hospital setting.

Taking a small rural community hospital and developing an outpatient surgical team could potentially take care of 65% of the general, orthopedic, ENT, and ophthalmology surgical needs locally. This is in part what is being done through the University of North Dakota Rural Surgery Support Program. Several communities have reinvented a local surgical program that is for outpatient procedures only to include general surgery, orthopedics, and ophthalmology. Great care is made to properly screen patients so that they meet the criteria for an outpatient procedure and that there are proper local resources for the postoperative rehabilitation very similar to what is being done in the "big" cities.

SUMMARY

The scope of practice of the rural surgeon depends not only on the ability and training of the surgeon, but also the characteristics of the community served, community resources, geographic barriers, staff, money, local "ground rules." For anyone interested in the practice of rural surgery, one must read Dr Chester B. McVay's Presidential Address to the Central Surgical Association from 1962.[11] As a matter of introduction, Dr McVay left the big city academic world to practice and teach in Yankton, South Dakota, in the 1950s until his death in 1987. He was the only surgeon for more than 100,000 rural citizens of South Dakota, Iowa, and Nebraska. His scope of practice was very diverse, which obviously entailed detailed work on hernia repair. In that address he stated, "Every hospital with a well-trained general surgeon cannot handle all types of surgery but the great bulk of the available surgery falls within the scope of the general surgeon." He later stated that, "Special problems outside the experience of a given surgeon can readily be referred. However, the general surgeon who is in a community without the ancillary specialties *must* be proficient in all phases of surgery from the standpoint of the acute emergencies. This includes the surgery of trauma in all of its phases and the diagnostic acumen to manage the emergency creditably."

In 1994, Donaldson and colleagues[12] defined primary care as "the provision of integrated, accessible health care services by clinicians who are accountable for addressing a large majority of personal health care needs, developing a sustained partnership with patients, and practicing in the context of family and community." In reality, the rural surgeon, or should we say, the surgeon who practices in a geographically isolated area, has to have all of those characteristics of primary care and one more—he or she must be able to operate with the skill set specific for the community needs.

DISCLOSURE

The author has no disclosures of any financial or commercial conflicts of interest.

REFERENCES

1. Cogbill TH, Bintz M. Rural General Surgery. A 38-year experience with a regional network established by an integrated health system in the mid-western United States. J Am Coll Surg 2017;02:115–22.
2. Landercasper J, Bintz M, Cogbill TH, et al. Spectrum of general surgery in rural America. Arch Surg 1997;132:494–6.
3. Harris JD, Hosford CC, Sticca RP. A comprehensive analysis of surgical procedures in rural surgery practices. Am J Surg 2010;200:820–5.
4. Anderson RL, Anderson MA. Rural general surgery: a review of the current situation and realties from a rural community practice in central Nebraska. Online J Rural Res Policy 2012;07(2):1–19.
5. Perl VU, Diggs B, Ham B, et al. Does surgery residency prepare residents to work at critical access hospitals? Am J Surg 2015;209:828–33.
6. Puls MW. Improving access to surgical care in rural America: an interview with J. David Richardson. Bull 2015;10:1–3.
7. Deal SB, Cook MR, Hughes D, et al. Training for a career in rural and nonmetropolitan surgery—a practical needs assessment. J Surg Educ 2018;75:229–33.
8. Cook MR, Hughes D, Deal SB, et al. When rural is no longer rural: demand for subspecialty trained surgeons increases with increasing population of a nonmetropolitan area. Am J Surg 2019;218:1022–7.
9. Steiner CA, Karaca Z, Moore BJ, et al. Surgeries in hospital-based ambulatory surgery and hospital inpatient settings. 2014. Available at: https://www.hcup-us.ahrq.gov/reports/statbriefs/sb223-Ambulatory-Inpatient-Surgeries-2014.jsp. Accessed May 1, 2017.
10. Imran JB, Madni TD, Taveras LU, et al. Analysis of operating room efficiency between a hospital-owned ambulatory surgical center and hospital outpatient department. Am J Surg 2019;218:809–12.
11. McVay CB. Surgery in the Rural Midwest. Arch Surg 1962;85:23–31.
12. Donaldson M, Yordy K, Vanselow N, editors. Defining primary care: an interim report. Washington, DC: National Academy Press; 1992.

Status of the Rural Surgical Workforce

John Patrick Walker, MD

KEYWORDS

- Rural surgery • Rural medical workforce • Rural healthcare shortages
- Rural surgery education

KEY POINTS

- Surgeons are critical to the survival of the rural hospital. They provide stabilization of trauma (and often definitive care), cancer screening, diagnosis, and nonoperative management of digestive diseases as well as numerous surgical procedures.
- The existence of the rural general surgeon is threatened by a lack of medical students from a rural areas and rural-specific surgical training as well as an aging population of general surgeons out in the community.
- The rural general surgeon is a substantial part of the economy of the community, generating 26 jobs, $1.4 million in payroll, and $2.7 million in revenue.
- It is imperative that existing surgical residencies develop rural surgical training tracts to supply a workforce to the 60 million rural Americans. Curriculums have been developed that can be instituted by almost all academic centers.
- Solutions to the rural surgical workforce include educating rural youth on the pathway of becoming a physician; development of science, technology, engineering, and mathematics programs in rural America; prioritizing recruitment of college students from rural areas to medical schools; providing financial aid for rural students in medical school; selection of medical students with a rural background to surgical residencies; and the development of rural tract within existing residency programs.

THE SURGEON IS THE CRITICAL COMPONENT FOR SURVIVAL OF RURAL HOSPITALS

Without a doubt the surgeon is the lynchpin in delivery of comprehensive health care in rural areas. A well-trained surgeon can provide basic health care, cancer screening, and trauma stabilization (and in many cases definitive care) as well as solid general surgery—from biopsies to hernias to gallbladders. Without addressing the shortage of surgeons in these areas, rural populations soon will find themselves traveling further and receiving acute care in a delayed fashion; in truth, they will become second class citizens from a health care perspective. From a surgical viewpoint, the lack of a surgeon directly affects the delivery of trauma care, with injuries more likely to be fatal

Department of Surgery, The University of Texas Medical Branch, 301 University Boulevard, Galveston, TX 77555-0527, USA
E-mail address: jopwalke@UTMB.edu

Surg Clin N Am 100 (2020) 869–877
https://doi.org/10.1016/j.suc.2020.06.006
0039-6109/20/

for rural residents than for urban ones.[1] It appears to be a lack of specialists rather than a lack of primary care providers that is associated with higher mortalities in rural Medicare beneficiaries.[2] This article addresses numbers, qualifications, and recommendations to provide for an adequate rural surgical workforce.

GENERAL SURGEONS ARE IN SHORT SUPPLY

The number of Americans living in rural areas is approximately 60 million. Despite a lesser percentage of patients living in rural areas, the absolute number has remained stable for decades. In 2013, there were 28,190 general surgeons in the United States. In 2025, there will be approximately 30,760 general surgeons with a demand for 33,730—a need for 2970 more general surgeons. For all the 10 surgical specialties combined, there will be an estimated 20,340 full-time equivalents short.[3] There are approximately 2000 rural general surgeons; but in truth it is not really known exactly how many there are and the nature of their practice.[4]

THE RURAL GENERAL SURGEON

At present, 8% of surgeons are caring for the 20% of the population living in a rural area.[5] The rural surgeon is older (50–55 years) and mostly male, with 60% planning to retire in the next 10 years. Unfortunately, the number of rural surgeons continues to decline. There are multiple reasons for this phenomenon: the perception that rural surgeons have less diagnostic capabilities and modern equipment, the burden of call, training with a team concept of delivery, and most importantly—a decline in medical students and residents who have lived in, or studied in, a rural area. Although it is true that most rural hospitals do not have the equipment/facilities of the urban hospitals, many procedures performed by rural surgeons do not require much of a physical plant. Endoscopy and laparoscopy equipment, ultrasound, computerized tomography, and safe anesthesia allow for the performance of most procedures. Call is a problem—without a doubt it takes a special individual to take call every other day or even every day. There must be a dedication and love for the specialty and patients that are of the highest commitment. In today's world of "work-life balance" and wellness, rural surgeons must feel that their own wellness is best provided for by the satisfaction of caring for their patients. Likewise, the provision of health care by a comprehensive team (particularly in oncology and trauma) is going to be different in the rural setting. The team will likely include nurses, Certified Registered Nurse Anesthetists, and family practitioners. Their lack of focused training in a specific field of medicine often can be offset by their commitment to their hometown. In addition, compensation is a real challenge. Rural areas have a higher level of poverty, a larger percentage of Medicare beneficiaries,[6] and no backstop hospital for the needy to go to for definitive care. The rural surgeon likely is practicing in a critical access facility with limited funds to acquire the newest equipment. Nonetheless, that hospital probably is the second largest employer in the county (behind the school district) and providing high-paying jobs—supporting the already compromised rural economies.[7] The general surgeon is a substantial part of this economy, generating $2.7 million in revenue, $1.4 million in payroll, and 26 jobs.[8] And when a hospital loses its general surgeon, it has a much higher chance of closure. In hospitals that close, the average decrease in general surgeons was 6.9% in the 4 years before closure and 8.3% in the year before closure: "...this supports the theory that physician supply-especially the supply of surgeons-is a key determinant of hospital viability."[9] Seven percent of US counties lost their general surgeon from 2006 to 2011.[10]

WHO ARE THE RURAL PHYSICIANS?

Although some medical schools and residencies are developing rural tracts, there still is a gross discrepancy in the number of students from rural America. (Many of the osteopathic schools are developing rural tracts, but the allopathic schools are lagging.) One thing is for sure: a majority of physicians practicing in a rural setting were exposed to life in the country at some point—they grew up there, they went to college there, or they had a rural rotation as a medical student or resident.[11–13] Factors associated with rural surgical practice included attending a nonurban high school ($P = .001$) or college ($P = .001$), having a spouse/partner who grew up in a nonurban area ($P = .022$), and an interest in hunting birds ($P = .010$) or large game ($P = .001$). Those choosing rural practice were more likely than their urban counterparts to have completed a rural clerkship during medical school (79% vs 37%, respectively; $P = .001$).[14] General surgeons who were raised in a rural environment report that they are residing and practicing in a rural setting.[15] Of great concern is that at the present time only 5% of medical students come from a rural background.[16] There is some evidence that exposing an urban student to a rural practice may influence them to become a rural practitioner.[17]

THE DILEMMA

So, the dilemma—11% of physicians practice in a rural area compared with a rural population of 20% of the country,[18] and the medical schools are graduating only 5% of their class with a likelihood of practicing in the country. This is compounded by the fact that rural Americans have higher rates of chronic illness and less access to preventative medical care.[19,20] Further reducing the potential for medical students practicing in rural areas is that current medical students are showing less interest in rural medicine.[21] A survey by Merritt Hawkins in 2017 showed that only 3% of residents would consider practicing in a town of less than 25,000.[22] The number of physician assistants and nurse practitioners is predicted to double by 2030.[23] This increase in advanced practitioners could (if they are trained in endoscopy) reduce the cases available for the rural surgeon (and make it harder to recruit/obtain one).

SOLUTIONS

There are multiple solutions to the rural physician workforce shortage. These include educating rural youth in the pathway to become a physician, assistance with developing science programs in rural schools, and, of course, financial aid for rural students in medical school. Most rural hospitals assist with or assume student debt to recruit a new physician, especially a surgeon. Rural students' parents tend to have attained a lower level of education themselves and may be unequipped to give guidance to their children.[24] It is imperative that part of the solution is to reach out to rural high school students to show them the pathway to become a physician. Rural surgeons must be part of this. Although hospital administrators increasingly are concerned with allowing students to observe in the operating room, they must be brought to understand that without an early commitment to youth, the pipeline of future surgeons will dry up. There is no stronger influence than a visit to the operating room to enlighten a high school student that surgery is their future.

TRAINING THE RURAL SURGEON

It is imperative that organized surgery support the growth of rural training tracts. When looking at the current emphasis on rural training by specialties that might practice in a rural area, the surgical specialists are performing poorly. In a recent study of 1849 residency programs in anesthesiology, emergency medicine, general surgery, internal medicine, obstetrics and gynecology, pediatrics, and psychiatry, only 119 (6%) were rurally located or offered a rural track.[25] Only 36 programs require at least 8 weeks of rural training for some or all residents. In 2009, only 25 general surgery residency programs meet at least 1 of 3 criteria that might define a rural training program: a rural location, a rural-focused curriculum, or a self-identified interest in rural training.[26] The American College of Surgeons Web site section on education lists only 14 programs that have a special focus on rural surgery. Many residents completing general surgery training feel ill prepared to practice in a rural area.[27] Some surgeons feel that a rural tract should involve rural rotations. Although some exposure to a community hospital is necessary, the skills needed to be a competent rural surgeon can be found within any academic program. A rural practice is quite varied. Rural surgeons average 1071 procedures/year, composed of 25.6% general surgery, 39.8% endoscopy, 17.9% minor surgery, and 12.3% surgical specialty procedures.[28] In addition to the cases/subject manner required by the American Board of Surgery, rural surgeons should have skills in plastic surgery/hand, urology, gynecology (to include cesarean sections), orthopedics (especially nonoperative management/stabilization) otolaryngology, and interventional radiology[29] (**Box 1**). Because, almost certainly, they will be the gastroenterologist for their rural area, they must be an expert in endoscopy. At the University of Texas Medical Branch in Galveston, the addition of medical mission trips is a useful adjunct that can help prepare the resident for a rural practice (Keyan Mobli, Rece Laney, and Lauren Mctaggart, Medical Mission trips as an adjunct to surgical residency training, personal communication, 2020). Without a doubt a dedicated rural training tract increases the likelihood that a resident will practice in a similar setting.[30]

CRITICAL ACCESS HOSPITALS

The year 2019 was the worst for US rural hospital closures in a decade, with 19 hospital closures.[31] Almost all rural hospitals must become critical access hospitals (CAHs) to survive in today's environment. This allows for cost-based reimbursement rather than receiving compensation on a prospective payment system. Qualifications to be a CAH include 24/7 emergency service, a distance of 35 miles from another hospital, and having no more than 25 beds[32]; 28% of CAHs have operating rooms but no surgeons. Another requirement that can affect surgeons is a current limitation of 96 hours for admitted patients (although legislation currently is being considered to remove this rule). This certainly will dissuade rural surgeons from taking care of significantly ill patients and may make the job less desirable for some surgeons.

QUALITY OF RURAL SURGERY

One of the significant problems facing the rural surgeon is the feeling that volume equals quality. Although this may be true for some specific procedures (such as pancreatectomy and esophagectomy), rural surgeons have been shown to produce results in many areas very similar to their urban colleagues. The 2015 report of the Rural Health Research Center at the University of Washington, Seattle, showed that for a variety of common general surgery, obstetrics and gynecology, and orthopedic procedures, patients treated in rural hospitals had fewer serious complications than their urban counterparts, although the rural hospital cohort appeared to be less complex.[33] Gadzinski and colleagues[34] compared results from 1283 CAHs and 3612 non-CAHs for 8 common procedures in general surgery, obstetrics and gynecology, and

Box 1
Recommended curriculum for training a rural surgeon

General surgery—to include the required casework of the American Board of Surgery with emphasis on

Gastrointestinal endoscopy, including percutaneous gastrostomy, thyroidectomy, parathyroidectomy, benign and malignant breast conditions, laparoscopic and open common bile duct exploration, evaluation of gastroesophageal reflux disease and laparoscopic antireflux procedures, gastrectomy, laparoscopic appendectomy, laparoscopic inguinal and ventral hernia, laparoscopic colectomy, adrenalectomy, soft tissue tumors including sarcoma, management of melanoma, and sentinel node biopsy

Trauma

Advanced trauma life support protocol, including definitive and temporizing management of all traumatic injuries, burn management, and stabilization of trauma

Obstetrics/gynecology

Cesarean section, hysterectomy, oophorectomy, ovarian cysts and ectopic pregnancy, posterior(rectocele) repair, dilation and curettage, and rectovaginal fistula

Urology

Cystoscopy, retrogrades, placement of ureteral stents, percutaneous nephrostomy, management of bladder outlet obstruction in male patients, cystostomy tubes, neoureterostomy, psoas hitch, nephrectomy

Orthopedics

Closed management of fractures and dislocations, pelvic and spinal fracture management, basic hand surgery for trauma and infection, and amputations

Thoracic

Chest tubes, thoracentesis, pleurodesis, tracheostomy, video-assisted thoracoscopic surgery, thoracotomy with lobectomy and pneumonectomy, sternotomy, flexible and rigid bronchoscopy, mediastinoscopy, pericardial window, esophagectomy, management of ruptured esophagus (stent and open), chest trauma, and rib stabilization

Plastics

Skin grafts, common flaps, and tissue expanders (ie, for breast augmentation)

Interventional radiology

Ultrasound-guided biopsy, basic bedside and intraoperative duplex/ultrasound, fluoroscopic techniques and radiation safety, computed tomography and fluoroscopically guided biopsy and drain placement, stereotactic breast biopsy with clip or needle placement, radioisotope assisted sentinel node biopsy, foregut and hindgut contrast imaging, and laparoscopic common bile duct imaging

Ear, nose, and throat

Tonsillectomy and adenoidectomy, bilateral myringotomy and tubes, excision of salivary glands, diagnosis and management of head and neck cancer, drainage of peritonsillar abscess, extraction of foreign bodies, management of refractory epistaxis, and evaluation of facial trauma

Vascular

Ruptured abdominal aortic aneurysm, embolectomy, bypass, or shunt placement for acute limb ischemia, management of acute venous thrombotic disease, inferior vena cava filter placement, mesenteric ischemia evaluation and treatment options, management of compartment syndrome and reperfusion syndrome, fasciotomy, hemodialysis access, management of peripherally inserted central catheter lines, mediports, diagnostic and basic interventional angiographic techniques, thrombolytic techniques, carotid endarterectomy, balloon angioplasty and basic stenting techniques, prosthetic and autogenous bypass procedures, and venous ablative procedures for lower extremity varicosities

Guidelines

It is imperative that the rural surgeon be taught the importance of evidence-based medicine and following guidelines—such as the National Comprehensive Cancer Network recommendations for cancer care. If practicing in a rural area, following national recommendations ensures quality of care.

orthopedics. These included appendectomy, cholecystectomy, colorectal cancer resection, cesarean section, hysterectomy, knee replacement, hip replacement, and surgical repair of hip fractures.[34] Except for hip fracture in Medicare beneficiaries, length of stay was shorter at CAHs for 4 procedures and mortality rates were equivalent. Ibraham and colleagues[35] retrospectively reviewed 1,631,904 admissions and published an analysis of surgical outcomes and expenditures among Medicare beneficiaries treated in 828 CAHs and 3676 non-CAHs. Four common general surgery procedures were included: appendectomy, cholecystectomy, colectomy, and hernia repair. The investigators noted that among Medicare beneficiaries undergoing common surgical procedures, patients admitted to CAHs compared with non-CAHs had no significant difference in 30-day mortality rates, serious complication rates, and lower Medicare expenditures, but had fewer medical comorbidities.[35] So, at least for some common procedures, results in a rural hospital are competitive with urban facilities. It might not even matter. When faced with a higher complication rate of having a surgery at a rural hospital, the elderly still rwould rather have their surgery near home.[36]

NO NEED FOR SUBSPECIALIZATION

Another factor in obtaining surgeons for the rural workforce is that 77% of residents are pursuing subspecialization,[37] when the job market for general surgeons actually is greater than that for specialty trained surgeons. In a report by Decker and colleagues,[38] 46% of job offerings were for rural surgeons and do not require additional training. Fellowship training was required for 18%, 28%, and 92% of jobs posted for rural, nonacademic, and academic postings, respectively. Unless they are interested in academics, by subspecializing, trainees may be taking themselves out of the market, rather than becoming more marketable. A survey of rural hospital administrators showed that 34% of rural hospitals have a surgeon leaving within the next 2 years and more than one-third of rural hospitals were searching for a general surgeon.[39]

WHAT NEEDS TO BE DONE NOW

In summary (paraphrasing Henry and colleagues[40]), to increase the number of rural surgeons, the pipeline must be increased: (1) structured contact between rural high school students and the medical profession; (2) selection of rural students into medical schools; (3) rural exposure during medical training; (4) selection of rural students into surgical training; (4) rural tracts in surgical training; and (5) a concerted effort to attract and retain rural general surgeons. Elements to enhance the success of these include having rural practitioners on selection committees for medical school and residencies. Certainly, financial incentives for rural surgeons to take medical students and residents would move more surgeons out "into the country."

WHAT NEEDS TO BE DONE NOW

The Crisis is here—the loss of rural surgeons leads to the loss of rural hospitals. The citizens lose access to care, which in truth places them in the same category as the uninsured and the poor. These largely are older patients who do not have access to care. Access to health care is a right that should be provided to all citizens, in particular, those who live in the heartland—rural Americans. The time to act is now—all of us must work to produce more broadly trained surgeons who can and will practice in the rural environment.

DISCLOSURE

The author has nothing to disclose.

REFERENCES

1. Jarman MP, Castillo RC, Carlini AR, et al. Rural risk: geographic disparities in trauma mortality. Surgery 2016;160(6):1551–9.
2. Johnston KJ, Wen H, Joynt Maddox KE. Lack of access to specialists associated with mortality and preventable hospitalizations of rural medicare beneficiaries. Health Aff (Millwood) 2019;38(12):1993–2002.
3. U.S. Department of Health and Human Services, Health Resources and Services Administration, National Center for Health Workforce Analysis. 2016. National and regional projections of supply and demand for surgical specialty practitioners 2013- 2025. Rockville (MD).
4. Mahoney ST, Strassle PD, Schroen AT, et al. Survey of the US Surgeon Workforce: Practice Characteristics, Job Satisfaction, and Reason for Leaving Surgery. J Am Coll Surg 2020;230(3):283–93.e1.
5. Puls MW. Shortage of rural surgeons: How bad is it? Bull Am Coll Surg 2018; 105(4):52–5.
6. Rural Health Information Hub. Social determinants of health for rural people. 2019. Available at: https://wwwruralhealthinfo.org/topics/social-determinants-of-health. Accessed July 13, 2020.
7. Doeksen GA, Cordes S, Shaffer R. Health care's contribution to rural economic development. Stillwater (OK): National Center for Rural Health Works, Oklahoma State University, Oklahoma Cooperative Extension; 1992.
8. Eilrich FC, Sprague JC, Whitacre BE, et al. The economic impact of a rural general surgeon and model for forecasting need. Stillwater (OK): National Center for Rural Health Works, Oklahoma State University, Oklahoma Cooperative Extension; 2010.
9. Germack HD, Kandrack R, Martself GR. When rural hospitals close, the physician workforce goes. Health Aff (Millwood) 2019;38(12):2086–94.
10. Nakayama DK, Hughes TG. Issues that face rural surgery in the United States. J Am Coll Surg 2014;219(4):814–8.
11. Rabinowitz HK, Diamond JJ, Markham FW, et al. The relationship between entering medical students' background and career plans and their rural practice outcomes three decades later. Acad Med 2012;87(4):493–7.
12. Pretorius RW, Lichter MI, Okazaki G, et al. Where do they come from and where do they go: implications of geographic origins of medical students. Acad Med 2010;85(10 Suppl):S17–20.
13. Owen JA, Conaway MR, Bailey BA, et al. Predicting rural practice using different definitions to classify medical school applicants as having a rural upbringing. J Rural Health 2007;23(2):133–40.
14. Jarman BT, Cogbill TH, Mathiason MA, et al. Factors correlated with surgery resident choice to practice general surgery in a rural area. J Surg Educ 2009;66(6): 319-324.
15. Doty B, Heneghan S, Gold M, et al. Is a broadly-based surgical residency program more likely to place graduates in rural practice? World J Surg 2006; 30(12):2089–93 [discussion: 2094].
16. Shipman SA, Wendling A, Jones KC, et al. The decline in rural medical students: a growing gap in geographic diversity threatens the rural physician workforce. Health Aff (Millwood) 2019;38(12):2011–9.

17. Tolhurst HM, Adams J, Stewart SM. An exploration of when urban background medical students become interested in rural practice. Rural Remote Health 2006;6:452.
18. Fordyce MA, Chen FM, Doescher MP, et al. 2005 physician supply and distribution in rural area of the United States. Seattle (WA): University of Washington Rural Health Research Center; 2007. Available at: https://depts.washington.edu/uwrhrc/uploads/RHRC%20FR116%20Fordyce.pdf. Accessed July 13, 2020.
19. Dwyer-Lindgren L, Bertozzi-Villa A, Stubbs RW, et al. Inequalities in Life Expectancy among US counties 1980 – 2014: temporal trends and key drivers. JAMA Intern Med 2017;177(7):1003–11.
20. Casey MM, Thiede CF, Klingner JM, et al. Are Rural residents less likely to obtain recommended preventative healthcare services? Am J Prev Med 2001;21(3): 182–8.
21. Shipman SA, Jones KC, Erickson CE, et al. Exploring the workforce implications of a decade of medical school expansion: variations in medical school growth and changes in student characteristics and career plans. Acad Med 2013; 88(12):1904–12.
22. 2017 Survey: Final-year medical resident. Merritt Hawkins. Available at: www.merritthawkins.com/uploadedFiles/mha_resident_survey.pdf. Accessed July 13, 2020.
23. Association of American Medical Colleges. The complexities of physician supply and demand: Projections from 2015-2030. Available at: https://aamc-black.global.ssl.fastly.net/production/media/filer_public/a5/c3/a5c3d565-14ec-48fb947b-99fafaeech00aamc_projections_update_2017.pdf. Accessed July 13, 2020.
24. Torpey E. Measuring the value of education. Washington (DC): Bureau of labor statistics; 2018. Available at: https://www.bis.gov/carreeroutlook/2018/data-ondisplay/education-pays.htm. Accessed July 13, 2020.
25. Patterson DG, Andrilla CHA, Garberson LA. Preparing physicians for rural practice: availability of rural training in rural-centric residency programs. J Grad Med Educ 2019;11(5):550–7.
26. Doty B, Zuckerman R, Borgstrom D. Are general surgery residency programs likely to prepare future rural surgeons? J Surg Educ 2009;66(2):74–9.
27. Gillman LM, Vergis A. General surgery graduates may be ill prepared to enter rural or community surgical practice. Am J Surg 2013;205(6):752–7.
28. Harris JD, Hosford CC, Sticca RP. A comprehensive analysis of surgical procedures in rural surgery practices. Am J Surg 2010;200(6):820–5.
29. Sticca RP, Mullin BC, Harris JD, et al. A comprehensive analysis of surgical procedures in rural surgery practices. Am J Surg 2012;204(6):1007–12.
30. Deveney K, Deatherage M, Oehling D, et al. Association Between Dedicated Rural Training Year and the Likelihood of Becoming a General Surgery in a Small Town. JAMA Surg 2013;148(9):817–21.
31. Available at: https://www.theguardian.com/us-news/2020/feb/19/us-rural-hospital-closures-report. Accessed July 13, 2020.
32. Centers for Medicare and Medicaid Services. Critical Access Hospitals. Available at: https://www.gov/Outreach-and-Education/Medicare-LEarning-Network-MLN/MLNProducts/downloads/CritAccessHospfctsht.pdf. Accessed July 13, 2020.
33. Doescher MP, Jackson JE, Fordyce MA, et al. Variability in general surgical procedures in rural and urban U.S. hospital inpatient settings. Final Report #142. WWAMI Rural Health Research Center. Seattle (WA): University of Washington; 2015.

34. Gadzinski AJ, Dimick JB, Ye Z, et al. Utilization and outcomes of inpatient surgical care at critical access hospitals in the United States. JAMA Surg 2013;148(7): 589–96.
35. Ibraham AM, Hughes TG, Thumma JR, et al. Association of hospital critical access status with surgical outcomes and expenditures among Medicare beneficiaries. JAMA 2016;315(19):2095–103.
36. Finlayson SR, Birkmeyer JD, Tosteson AN, et al. Patient preferences for location of care: Implications for regionalization. Med Care 1999;37(2):204–9.
37. Borman KR, Vick LR, Biester TW, et al. Changing demographics of residents choosing fellowships: longterm data from the american board of surgery. J Am Coll Surg 2008;206(5):782–8.
38. Decker MR, Bronson NW, Greenberg CC, et al. The general surgery job market: analysis of current demands for general surgeons and their specialized skills. J Am Coll Surg 2013;217(6):1133–9.
39. Doty B, Zuckerman R, Finlayson S, et al. General Surgery at rural hospitals: A national survey of rural hospital administrators. Surgery 2008;143(5):599–606.
40. Henry J, Edwards B, Crotty B. Why do medical graduates choose rural careers? Rural Remote Health 2009;9:1083.

Rural Standards and the Quality Equation

Michael Duke Sarap, MD[a,b,c,d,e,f,g,*]

KEYWORDS

- Rural surgery • Quality measurement
- American College of Surgeons quality programs • Accreditation • NSQIP

KEY POINTS

- Rural surgeons encounter barriers to measuring and documenting the quality of the care they provide in their local facilities.
- There are specific definitions of Quality and Value related to health care that can be used to identify areas for improvement.
- Several surgical standards programs and quality resources are available to surgeons to help measure, analyze, and benchmark their quality of surgical care, even in resource-limited environments.
- There are several definite advantages to patients, their families, and the US health care system that can be realized by keeping appropriate patients in local facilities for their care.

INTRODUCTION

There are 60 million people living in rural America, which represents 25% of the population yet only 10% of General Surgeons practice in those areas. Rural patients tend to be older, sicker, less educated, and economically disadvantaged. Rural areas have a higher prevalence of chronic diseases including heart disease and cancer. Rural residents tend to be less healthy than urban dwellers, in part because of lifestyle choices including higher rates of cigarette smoking, hypertension, and obesity and less physical activity.[1] Rural patients present with more advanced cancers than their urban counterparts. Specific rural regions, including Appalachia, have documented higher cancer incidences and mortality rates.[2] There are several barriers involved in providing surgical care for rural populations. These barriers include poor access to health care

The author has no disclosures.
[a] SE Med Department of Surgery, Cambridge, OH, USA; [b] American College of Surgeons, Advisory Council for Rural Surgery; [c] Commission on Cancer Program in Ohio; [d] Department of Surgery, Wright State University Boonshoft School of Medicine, Dayton, OH, USA; [e] Lake Erie College of Medicine, Erie, PA, USA; [f] Physicians Assistant Program, Marietta College; [g] Tina Kiser Cancer Concern Coalition
* 100 Clark Court, Cambridge, OH 43725.
E-mail address: msarap@msn.com

https://doi.org/10.1016/j.suc.2020.05.010 surigcal.theclinics.com

services and specialists; geographic barriers preventing access to providers, services, and technology; minimal transportation options for disease screening and treatment; limited knowledge about cancer and other health issues resulting in low participation in screening, early detection, and healthy lifestyle choices; and prohibitive costs of care.[3,4] Haider and colleagues, in a 2013 JACS article, described multiple interconnected factors related to the patients, providers, and the system of care that contribute to racial disparities in surgical care and outcomes in the United States. The article clearly defines many of the barriers to providing high-quality surgical care to rural Americans.[5]

Several examples of suboptimal care for patients with cancer in rural area have appeared in professional journals and meetings and in the lay press. Examples of rural cancer care inadequacies include lower use of needle biopsy and sentinel lymph node biopsy techniques for patients with breast cancer[6–9]; significantly lower rates of radiation treatment after breast cancer lumpectomy[10,11]; lower rates of adequate lymph node retrieval and appropriate adjuvant chemotherapy and higher death rates in patients with colon cancer[3,12,13]; higher mastectomy rates and late-stage cancers in patients with breast cancer[14]; higher likelihood of discharge to skilled nursing facility instead of home in patients with colon cancer[15]; and other similar examples. These conclusions all come from academic centers through large database studies. It is rare to see data collected and reported by rural centers involving those surgeons actually caring for patients with cancer in rural area. In many of the cases, local workforce and resource limitations may explain the differences in care and outcomes. For example, if the nearest radiation facility is more than 100 miles away, then most women with breast cancer will choose mastectomy over lumpectomy or may not complete their radiation therapy after lumpectomy, to avoid the time and expense of travel for postoperative radiation therapy. Access to care by specialists is often limited in rural areas. Aboagye and others at the University of Pittsburgh documented a rural-urban disparity in the density of gastroenterologists, general surgeons, and radiation oncologists who traditionally provide colorectal cancer screening and treatment.[16]

A study done by Finlayson documented that nearly 100% of rural patients preferred to receive their care locally, especially if the local quality of care was the same as that at the larger distant hospital. In fact, nearly half of the patients polled would choose to remain local even if the mortality rate at the local hospital was double that of a hospital requiring the patient to travel for their surgical care.[17] More recent papers, however, suggest that patients may be bypassing their local hospitals for care because of concerns about the quality of the care provided locally.[3,18,19]

RURAL BARRIERS TO MEASURING THE QUALITY OF SURGICAL CARE

Rural and small community surgeons have certain barriers that prevent them from measuring, documenting, and publicizing the specifics of the care provided to their patients. These surgeons are often in single or small group practices and manage their own businesses. They have no office or hospital staff dedicated to quality endeavors. Financial and time constraints prevent them from being champions of quality surgical care in their communities. In addition, small numbers of specific cases can result in high statistical complication and mortality rates even if these events happen infrequently.[3,20–22] This inability to collect and assess the quality of their surgical care can lead to patient outmigration and even "tiering" by third-party payers that forces patients away from their hometown hospitals and providers using financial disincentives.

The US government has developed a Quality Payment Program (QPP), including a Merit-Based Incentive Payment System (MIPPS), that is woefully inadequate in measuring and defining surgical quality care and value. Measures such as immunizations, blood pressure control, diabetes control, and smoking cessation are important gauges of a patient's overall health but are unrelated to episodes of surgical care. They also do not provide the information surgeons need to improve care.[23]

DEFINING AND MEASURING QUALITY

The Institute of Medicine's (IOM) seminal report "Crossing the Quality Chasm" defined quality as "the degree to which health services for individuals and populations increases the likelihood of desired health outcomes and are consistent with current professional knowledge."[24] The IOM (currently renamed The National Academy of Medicine) viewed quality as consisting of 6 sentinel attributes: safety, timeliness, effectiveness, patient centeredness, efficiency, and care that is equitable.

Safe—Delivering health care that minimizes risks and harm to patients, including avoiding preventable injuries and reducing medical errors.

Effective—Providing services based on scientific knowledge and evidence-based guidelines.

Timely—Reducing delays in providing and receiving health care.

Efficient—Delivering health care in a manner that maximizes resource use and avoids waste.

Equitable—Delivering health care that does not differ in quality according to personal characteristics such as gender, race, ethnicity, geographic location, or socioeconomic status.

Patient centered—Providing care that takes into account the preferences and aspirations of individual service users and the culture of their community.

Individuals and groups attempting to understand the quality of the care delivered to patients and populations should be investigating metrics of performance that reflect these 6 attributes.

The Institute for Healthcare Improvement later translated the IOM aims into a framework for action, the Triple Aim, consisting of better patient outcomes, improved patient satisfaction, and lower costs. The addition of physician and health care professional well-being expands the concept to The Quadruple Aim.

There are defined processes to facilitate measurement of the 6 aims including the following:

- Accreditation and Certification of Hospitals and Community-Based Services
- Clinical Quality Performance Measurement and Improvement
- Patient Safety Assurance and Harm Prevention
- Patient Experiences and Perceptions of Care[25,26]

Accreditation and/or Certification programs establish the basis for providing quality in health care. Accreditation is the foundation on which health care is delivered, but it is not a measure of quality, per say. It is more about how well an institution has performed in the past and how well the infrastructure for providing quality health care has been established. Clinical performance metrics are regarded as the ultimate measures of clinical quality. Process measures assess what and how care is provided and the appropriateness of care. Outcomes measures demonstrate how well care is provided and, potentially, the cost-benefits of the care.

Performance improvement over time is also a measure of quality. Avoiding patient injury and/or harm is an important component of clinical performance. Patient experiences and perceptions of care are essential metrics of patient centeredness.[25]

National discussions have moved beyond just assessing quality and now focus on the "Value" of health care. The Value Equation states that

Value = appropriateness x quality / cost to the patient

From a population standpoint, the Value Equation might read as follows:

Value = health outcomes that matter to patients (quality) / costs of delivering these outcomes over time

HOW TO MEASURE AND DOCUMENT THE SAFETY AND EFFECTIVENESS OF RURAL SURGICAL CARE?

Rural and small practice surgeons must begin to take the lead in collecting, assessing, and reporting information about the care they provide for their communities. The American College of Surgeons (ACS) and other surgical specialty organizations offer a wide spectrum of accreditation and certification programs that can help smaller facilities measure and improve the quality and value of their surgical services. ACS National Surgical Quality Improvement Program (NSQIP) "Small and Rural" is a smaller more affordable version of the quality program that is used by many larger centers. "Small" is defined as any hospital that performs less than 1680 "ACS NSQIP eligible" cases per year. A hospital is considered "Rural" if its zip code is in a rural or small area as defined by Rural-Urban Commuting Area data from the University of Washington. The program measures local outcomes and allows comparisons to other facilities of various sizes. NSQIP does require clerical staff to extract information from the patient chart and download information into the database.[27] Large facilities participating in NSQIP have documented that it helps to prevent 250 to 500 complications per hospital per year, saves lives, and reduces costs.[28]

The ACS is involved in many specific quality programs including the Commission on Cancer (CoC) Accreditation, ACS Committee on Trauma Certification, National Accreditation Program for Breast Centers (NAPBC), Pediatric and Geriatric Accreditation Programs, and others (**Fig. 1**). The ACS Committee on Trauma (COT) offers several levels of certification from the smallest facility designation of level IV to the highest level I attained by tertiary and large academic centers. The trauma standards manual lists resources required to be certified at each level, appropriate to their size and staffing. The personnel and resource demands and level of commitment increase at each higher level of certification. The care of trauma patients, and indeed all patients, is significantly elevated in the communities participating in the COT program at every level of certification. Other programs and tools developed by the American College of Surgeons can be used to elevate the quality of surgical care in any size hospital, including the ACS Surgeon Specific Registry (SSR), Strong For Surgery, ACS Surgical Risk Calculator, and Non-Opioid Postoperative Pain Management resources. The SSR program facilitates surgeon participation in the QPP and MIPPS programs by providing a site for data submission on individual surgical cases and overall participation in quality initiatives.[29]

Smaller institutions with a single surgeon may not have the financial and staff resources to formally participate in these programs, but each surgeon can assess what types of cases represent most of their individual caseload, whether that is endoscopy, breast, hernia, or gastrointestinal cases, and find national benchmarks that can easily be measured in their institutions. Every endoscopy department can collect data on cecal intubation rates, colonoscopy withdrawal times, adequacy of preps, adenoma detection rates and appropriate indications, and follow-up intervals.[30–34]

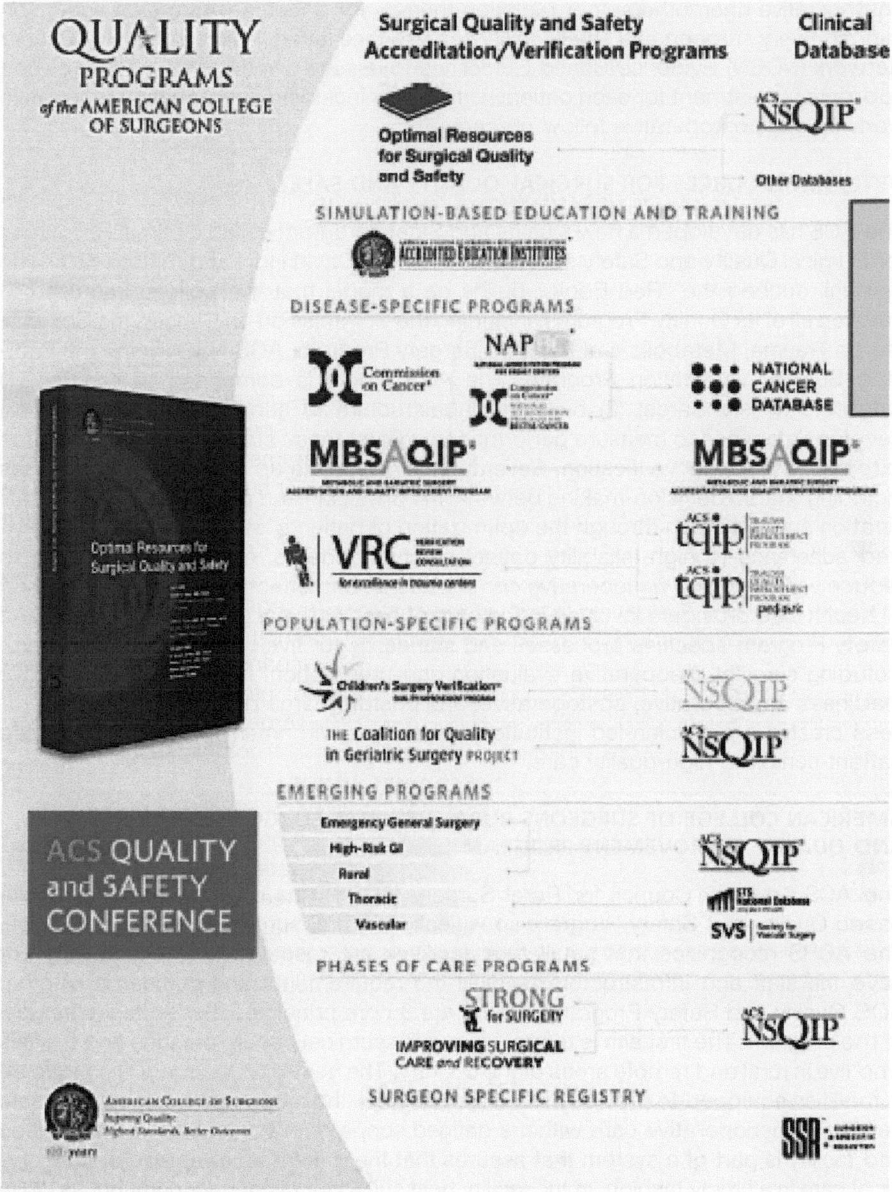

Fig. 1. American College of Surgeons quality and safety programs. (*Courtesy of* American College of Surgeons, Chicago, IL.)

Individual surgeons can pick and choose specific benchmarks from the NSQIP, Commission on Cancer, NAPBC, or ACS Committee on Trauma standards documents and use these to evaluate the care they provide.[29] Easy examples might include surgeon response time for highest level trauma activations, the number of lymph nodes harvested at colon cancer surgery, percentage of patients with breast cancer diagnosed with needle biopsy, and percentage treated with conservative surgery and appropriate postoperative chemotherapy or radiation therapy for patients with breast and colon cancer. Every surgeon and small facility can use the National Comprehensive Cancer Network (NCCN) Evidence-Based Guidelines to assess whether they have provided appropriate treatment for each patient with cancer including appropriate preoperative work-up and postoperative follow-up care.[35]

OPTIMAL RESOURCES FOR SURGICAL QUALITY AND SAFETY

The ACS has developed a new Quality and Safety program called Optimal Resources for Surgical Quality and Safety spearheaded by Drs David Hoyt and Clifford Ko.[36] The manual, dubbed the "Red Book," builds on a model that the College has used to develop all of its Quality Programs, including the Commission on Cancer, the Committee on Trauma, Metabolic and Bariatric Surgery Program, ACS NSQIP, and the Pediatric Surgery Verification Program. The ACS model is composed of 4 parts: (1) establish the standards; (2) build the infrastructure to support the standards; (3) develop databases to measure performance against those standards; and (4) provide external peer-review verification. Several principles make up the core of the process including shared decision-making between the physician and patient/family, risk stratification and reduction through the optimization of patients before surgery, standardized adherence to high-reliability patient-safety standards, evidence-based care to reduce variability and perioperative complications, and effective coordination among all health care providers involved in the care of each surgical patient. The Quality and Safety Program specifies processes and standards for five phases of surgical care, including surgical preoperative evaluation and preparation, immediate preoperative readiness, intraoperative, postoperative, and postdischarge phases of care. The process creates a physician-led institutional learning environment designed to provide patient-centered, high-quality care.[36]

AMERICAN COLLEGE OF SURGEONS RURAL HOSPITAL SURGICAL VERIFICATION AND QUALITY IMPROVEMENT PROGRAM

The ACS Advisory Council for Rural Surgery (ACRS) has developed a Red Book–based Quality and Safety Program specifically for rural surgeons and rural facilities. The ACRS recognizes that small rural facilities are resource limited and may not have the staff and infrastructure to fulfill the requirements and standards of other ACS Quality and Safety Programs. There are 3 core principles that underlie the goal of the program. The first aim is to provide quality surgical care to persons and families who live in rural and remote areas of the country. The next is that surgery is conducted in facilities equipped to provide essential personnel and infrastructure to support safe delivery of perioperative care within a defined scope of practice. Lastly, the surgeon and facility is part of a system that assures that the patient receives appropriate surgical care in a timely fashion, in the facility best suited for his or her condition, as close to his or home community as practicable. The Rural Surgery Standards Program focuses specifically on those surgical diseases and procedures that are common to most small hospitals and attempts to define those processes, resources, and infrastructure required to assure safe, high-quality care for surgical patients in smaller facilities. The standards define those resources and services required to support the care of the surgical patient, which include staffing and infrastructure in the emergency room; radiology, laboratory, pharmacy, and pathology services; nursing units including post-anaesthetic care unit, intensive care unit, and inpatient surgical units; and respiratory therapy and support staff in the operating room. Data collection and surveillance and data-driven quality improvement activities are the foundation of elevating the quality of the local care. The program also assures that those more complex surgical conditions that arrive at the smaller facility have well-defined protocols to properly resuscitate and transfer those patients to the appropriate tertiary facilities in the shortest amount of time.[37] In addition to improvements in quality and patient safety, participation in the Rural Surgery Standards Program can serve to elevate the reputation of the facility in their community, help local surgeons and administrators plan for appropriate resource and infrastructure improvements, and increase the probability of successful recruitment of new surgeons to the facility. Using a combination of already well-established surgical treatment standards, rural accreditation programs, and benchmarking local results against national results, rural surgeons can establish that their local care is indeed safe and effective for the vast number of surgical problems.

The manufacturing industry and businesses such as Motorola and General Electric have used other quality programs that have now been adapted to the health care sector. These types of programs include Six Sigma, Lean, and the Institute for Healthcare Improvement. Physicians are involved as Champion Sponsors and lead project teams. These programs are similar to the ACS Quality Programs in that they ask the organization to define, measure, analyze, improve, control, or Plan-Do-Study-Act.[38,39]

THE COST OF HEALTH CARE AND ITS EFFECT ON VALUE

The cost of health care, a key component of value, continues to increase and plays a major role in the goal of providing the most appropriate care for the patient. Much has been written about the significant numbers of medical care-related bankruptcies and especially the "financial toxicity" of cancer care. Nine of ten uninsured and one in ten privately insured patients with cancer are at risk of financial toxicity after their surgery.[40–43] Any calculation of cost should include the costs associated with travel to remote facilities for care and the costs to the patient's family for travel, meals, and lodging. A review article from the University of Iowa reports that more than 1.6 million rural households do not have cars, with higher rates of "carlessness" in the South, Appalachia, the Southwest, and Alaska.[44] Rural patients are affected by the financial toxicity of health care at higher rates than their urban counterparts.[45] Certain groups of individuals, such as the Amish population usually without phones or motorized transportation, are nearly impossible to care for outside their immediate areas. Social and economic costs are incurred with disruptions in family, work, and education schedules for treatment. A 2008 study revealed that patients in large rural towns must travel a median of 51 minutes to get to any specialized oncology care, those in even smaller towns travel 59 minutes and suffer even longer travel times of 83 and 97 minutes respectively to get to academic-based care.[46] Increased travel distance to a cancer facility negatively affects the likelihood that patients with stage II/III rectal cancer will receive radiation therapy to treat their disease.[47] A study by the nonprofit firm Altarum estimated that the time consumers spend waiting for or traveling to health care services costs $89 billion each year. Health care wait times are more than double wait times of other professional services.[48]

Lastly, treatment in a facility remote from the patient's hometown results in a lack of social support from family, friends, and social groups. Rural and socioeconomically challenged patients and families suffer the consequences of these hidden costs at a higher rate than their urban counterparts. Few of these factors have been well studied. Dr Nynikka Palmer and co-authors[49] at Wake Forest analyzed data from cancer survivors and found that patients aged 65 years or older were 66% more likely than their urban counterparts to forego medical care and 54% more likely to forego dental care because of cost. They noted that older cancer survivors in rural areas have to travel further to reach a medical provider, incurring greater out-of-pocket costs associated with travel and lost wages.[50] In ASCO's The State of Cancer Care in America: 2014, President Clifford Hudis, MD FACP stated that patient access to cancer care is directly tied to the survival of smaller, community practices. He states that people who are very sick, often elderly, with compromised immune systems and struggling with great fatigue and discomfort, traveling long distances for care is not just inconvenient, but potentially harmful.[50] Nathan and colleagues studied the excess expenditures incurred due to care at hospitals with substantially higher average costs than nearby facilities. They highlighted the potential for substantial savings by keeping patients in local low-cost facilities for their care.[51] Clearly, there are real medical, economic, and social advantages gained by caring for patients locally.

TIMELINESS OF CARE

Timeliness of care is also being studied across the spectrum of surgical care. Time to treat for patients with cancer has steadily lengthened over the last 2 decades. Median time to cancer treatment initiation increased significantly from 21 days in 2004 to 29 days in 2013. Dr Brian Bolwell, Chairman of the Cleveland Clinic Taussig Cancer Institute, addressed Time-To-Treat in a 2017 and 2019 Cleveland Clinic Cancer Advances Newsletter. For all cancer types, the larger the institution, the longer the wait time for patients, and the mean delay in 2017 was 43 days in US Comprehensive Cancer Centers.[52,53] Longer delays are associated with worsened overall survival for several cancer types depending on stage, including breast, lung, renal, pancreatic, and colon cancers. Delays of greater than 6 weeks were associated with substantially worsened survival.[53–56]

Tertiary centers are currently overburdened with complex patients, and wait times to transfer critically ill patients from smaller facilities can take several days. Many times the facilities are completely full and on diversion. The added burden of sending elective patients to remote centers that can receive high-quality care locally only adds to the wait times in big centers. Many studies predict a significant shortage of surgeons of all types by the year 2025. During this same time frame there will be a 43% increase in inpatient oncology surgeries and a 25% increase in outpatient cancer procedures. Experts predict that an additional 25% of cases now done by specialists will need to be done by general surgeons, many at the local centers, due to an insufficient surgical workforce.[57–59]

PATIENT CENTEREDNESS

Local patient care, if well organized and coordinated, is certainly patient-centered and can be very timely, cost-effective, and efficient. One could also argue that, because most of a rural surgeon's practice are friends, neighbors, and local community members, the care is very likely to be equitable. On average, Critical Access Hospitals have significantly higher ratings on HCAHPS measures than all US hospitals indicating high levels of patient satisfaction.[3,60]

More studies focusing on care in smaller facilities are required to document the quality of the local surgical care. The University of Michigan Center for Healthcare Outcomes and Policy has done multiple studies on the topic of surgical care in small rural facilities. Studies by Ibriham, Dimick, and others have documented that several common surgical procedures performed at small Critical Access Hospitals, including appendectomy, cholecystectomy, colectomy, and hernia repair, had the same 30-day mortality rates as larger hospitals, lower rates of serious complications, and lower costs as compared with larger hospitals. The patients from the smaller facilities also were less likely to be discharged to Skilled Nursing or Rehabilitation units.[61–63] Other studies involving small Critical Access Hospitals have documented rates of death, postoperative bleeding and hematoma, respiratory failure, deep vein thrombosis and pulmonary embolism, sepsis, and postoperative wound dehiscence that are the same or better than larger facilities.[64]

A significant amount of cancer care is delivered locally and much of it in nonaccredited facilities. Mary Charlton at the University of Iowa documented that nearly 40% of rural Iowans who are diagnosed with colorectal, breast, and lung cancer are being treated in hospitals that are not accredited by the Commission on Cancer.[65] Recognizing this rural disparity, the Commission on Cancer has formed an Interprogrammatic Task Force On Levels of Care along with the Breast and Rectal Accreditation Programs, the Medical (ASCO) and Radiation (ASTRO) Oncology groups, CoC State Chairs and Cancer Liaison Physicians, and the American Cancer Society. The goals are to (1) get the correct patient to the correct center for care, (2) optimize the delivery and outcomes of less complex care in a broader range of hospitals and programs (local care), and (3) engage the 943 nonmetro hospitals that are not Commission on Cancer Accredited.

The patient should be at the center of any discussion of the value of the care being provided. The National Comprehensive Cancer Network (NCCN), in a 2017 Policy Report, developed a definition of Value Tools for Patients. “A value tool for patients is a dynamic system, process or device that assists patients in articulating their personal preferences and goals with regards to their medical condition, treatment and related decision-making. These tools assist patients in communicating information to their providers, which in turn assists providers in delivering personalized care”. The principles of any tools developed include capturing patient preferences and values, ability to be incorporated into the care workflow, ability to personalize the tool to the specific needs of each individual patient during their treatment journey and life flow, and should be easily understandable and user friendly.[66] Although the NCCN group’s focus was on patients with cancer, this definition and any tools developed would be pertinent to any seriously ill surgical patient. An excellent example of a Value Tool would be the American College of Surgeons Surgical Risk Assessment Tool. Based on NSQIP data, the tool allows a surgeon to enter important clinical information about a specific patient and a planned surgical procedure, and the tool will calculate the chance of complications and death for that specific patient. An easily understood report can be printed out in color for the patient and patient’s family to facilitate a preoperative discussion about the risks, benefits, complications, and alternatives for the surgical procedure.[67]

SUMMARY

In summary, rural and small community surgeons must become quality leaders and local champions in assessing the quality and value of the surgical care being provided in their communities. There are significant burdens and barriers hindering accomplishment of this goal; however, there are significant numbers of resources and programs that can be used even in low-resource environments. Local care offers significant advantages to patients and their families in terms of cost, patient centeredness, patient support, efficiency of care, and other factors. Many small facilities already use these advantages and are measuring and benchmarking their local care against national standards and documenting the high quality and value of their locally provided care.

REFERENCES

1. Iglehart J. The challenging quest to improve rural health care. N Engl J Med 2018; 378:5.
2. Gosschalk A, Carozza S. Cancer in rural areas: a literature review. Rural Healthy People 2010. Available at: http://www.srph.tamhsc.edu/centers/rhp2010/Vol2cancer.htm. Accessed January 27, 2020.
3. Halverson A, Johnson J. Surgical quality and patient safety in rural settings. In: Sanchez JA, Barach P, Johnson P, et al, editors. Surgical patient care. Switzerland: Springer; 2017. Chapter 49.
4. Johnston KJ, Wen H, Maddox K. Lack of access to specialists associated with mortality and preventable hospitalizations of rural medicare beneficiaries. Health Aff 2019;38(No 12). Rural Health.
5. Haider A, Scott V, Rehman K, et al. Racial disparities in surgical care and outcomes in the United States. J Am Coll Surg 2013;216(No. 3):482–92.e12.
6. Gutwein L, Ang D, Liu H, et al. Utilization of minimally invasive breast biopsy for the evaluation of suspicious breast lesions. Am J Surg 2011;202(No. 2):127–32.
7. Adepoju L, Qu W, Kazan V, et al. The evaluation of national time trends, quality of care and factors affecting the use minimally invasive breast biopsy and open biopsy for diagnosis of breast lesions. Am J Surg 2014;208(3):382–90.
8. Zimmerman C, Sheffield K, Duncan C, et al. Time trends and geographic variation in use of minimally invasive breast biopsy. J Am Coll Surg 2013;216(4): 814–24 [discussion: 824–7].
9. Arrington A, Kruper L, Vito C, et al. Rural and urban disparities in the evolution of sentinel lymph node utilization in breast cancer. Am J Surg 2013;206(No. 5): 674–81.
10. Dickson-Witmer D, Bleznak A, Kennedy J, et al. Breast cancer care in the community: challenges, opportunities and outcomes. Surg Oncol Clin N Am 2011; 20:555–80.
11. Dragun A. Once-Weekly Breast Irradiation Following Lumpectomy Results in Better Compliance, Lower Costs and Comparable Cosmetic Outcomes vs daily Treatment, 2014 ASCO Breast Cancer Symposium, San Francisco (CA): September, 25-27.
12. Greenberg C, Lipsitz S, Neville B, et al. Receipt of appropriate surgical care for medicare beneficiaries with cancer. Arch Surg 2011;146(No. 10):1128–34.
13. Revels S, Wong S, Banerjee M, et al. Differences in perioperative care at low- and high-mortality hospitals with cancer surgery. Ann Surg Oncol 2014;21:2129–35.
14. Jethwa K. Breast cancer diagnosed at later stages in rural patients. American Association for Cancer Research Presentation; 2013.
15. Balentine C, Naik A, Robinson C, et al. Association of high-volume hospitals with greater likelihood of discharge to home following colorectal surgery. JAMA Surg 2014;149(No. 3):244–51.
16. Aboagye J, Kaiser H, Hayanga A. Rural-urban differences in access to specialist providers of colorectal cancer care in the US. JAMA Surg 2014;149(No 6): 537–43.
17. Finlayson S, Birkmeyer J, Tostenson J, et al. Patient preferences for location of care: implications for regionalization. Med Care 1999;37(No 2):204–9.
18. Williamson H, Hart LG, Pirani MJ, et al. Market shares for rural inpatient surgical services: where does the buck stop? J Rural Health 1994;10:70–9.
19. Liu J, Bellamy GR, McCormick M. Patient bypass behavior and critical access hospitals: implications for patient retention. J Rural Health 2007;23:17–24.

20. Nakayama D, Hughes T. Issues that face rural surgery in the United States. J Am Coll Surg 2014;219(No. 4):814–8.
21. Molt P. Rural Surgery and the Volume Dilemma. American College of Surgeons Bulletin. 2016. Available at: http://bulletin.facs.org/2016/10/rural-surgery-and-the-volume-dilemma/#.Wq5n22bMxo4. Accessed January 27, 2020.
22. O'Sullivan M. Safety in Numbers: Cancer Surgeries in California Hospitals. California Healthcare Foundation Report 2015. Available at: http://www.chcf.org/publications/2015/11/safety-cancer-surgeries-hospitals. Accessed January 27, 2020.
23. Zlatos C, Cofferon M, Opelka F, et al. Redefining Surgical Value in the Quality Payment Program. ACS Bulletin. 2019. Available at: http://bulletin.facs.org/2019/07/redefining-surgical-value-in-the-quality-payment-program/. Accessed January 27, 2020.
24. Crossing the quality Chasm: a new health system for the 21st 26 century. 2001. Available at: www.ncbi.nim.nih.gov/pubmed/25057539. Accessed January 27, 2020.
25. Cohen D. Quality in healthcare: a five-dimensional view. Patient safety and quality healthcare. 2012. Available at: https://www.psqh.com/analysis/quality-in-healthcare-a-five-dimensional-view/. Accessed January 27, 2020.
26. Wachter R, Gupta K. Understanding patient safety. 3rd edition. New York: McGraw-Hill Education; 2016.
27. American College of Surgeons National Surgical Quality Improvement Program (ACS NSQIP). Available at: www.acsnsqip.org. Accessed January 27, 2020.
28. Hall B, Barton H, Karen R, et al. Does Surgical Quality Improve in the American College of Surgeons NSQIP Program? Ann Surg 2009;250:363–76.
29. American College of Surgeons Quality Programs. Available at: https://www.facs.org/quality-programs. Accessed January 27, 2020.
30. Kaminski M, Regula J, Kraszewska E, et al. Quality indicators for colonoscopy and the risk of interval cancer. N Engl J Med 2010;362:1795–803.
31. Hsu C, Lin W, Su M, et al. Factors that influence cecal intubation rate during colonoscopy in deeply sedated patients. J Gastroenterol Hepatol 2012;27(No. 1):76–80.
32. Mehrotra A, Morris M, Gourevitch R, et al. Physician characteristics associated with higher adenoma detection rate. Gastrointest Endosc 2018;87:778–86.e5.
33. Pace D, Borgaonkar M, Evans B, et al. Annual colonoscopy volume and maintenance of competency for surgeons. Surg Endosc 2017;31:2630–5.
34. Bhangu A, Bowley D, Horner R, et al. Volume and accreditation, but not specialty, affect quality standards in colonoscopy. Br J Surg 2012;99:1436–44.
35. National Comprehensive Cancer Network (NCCN) Evidence Based Guidelines (NCCN.org).
36. Hoyt D, Ko C, editors. Optimal resources for surgical quality and safety. Chicago: American College of Surgeons; 2017. Available at: https://www.facs.org/quality-programs. Accessed January 27, 2020.
37. American College of Surgeons. Rural hospital surgical verification and quality improvement program manual. Chicago: ACS Advisory Council on Rural Surgery. American College of Surgeons Quality Programs; 2019. Available at: https://www.facs.org/quality-programs. Accessed January 27, 2020.
38. Varkey P, Reller M, Resar R. Basics of quality improvement in health care. Mayo Clin Proc 2007;82(No. 6):735–9.
39. Martin W., Quality Models: Selecting the Best Model to Deliver Results. William Marty Martin 2007:33.

40. Farooq A, Merath K, Hyer J, et al. Financial Toxicity Risk Among Adult Patients Undergoing Cancer Surgery in the US: An Analysis of the National Inpatient Sample. J Surg Oncol 2019. https://doi.org/10.1002/jso.25605.
41. Synder R, Chang G. Financial Toxicity: A Growing Burden For Cancer Patients. ACS Bulletin. 2019. Available at: https://bulletin.facs.org/2019/09/financial-toxicity-a-growing-burden-for-cancer-patients. Accessed January 27, 2020.
42. Center for Disease Control Morbidity and Mortality Report, June 13, 2014.
43. Mongelli M, Giri S, Peipert B, et al. Financial burden and quality of life among thyroid cancer survivors. J Surg 2019. https://doi.org/10.1016/j.surg.2019.11.014.
44. Charlton M, Schlichting J, Chioreso C, et al. Challenges of rural cancer care in the United States. Oncol J 2015;29(9):633–40.
45. Spencer J. Breast cancer takes heavier financial toll on black and rural women. J Natl Cancer Inst 2020;112(6):647–50.
46. Omega T. Geographic Access to Cancer Care in the US. Cancer 2008;112:909–18.
47. Linn C. Travel burden linked with likelihood of receiving radiation therapy to treat rectal cancer. Int J Radiat Oncol Biol Phys 2016;15:719–28.
48. Rhyan C. Travel and Wait Times are Longest for Health care Services and Result in an Annual Opportunity Cost of $89 Billion. Altarum Center for Value in Health Care. 2019. Available at: corwin.rhyan@altarum.org. Accessed January 27, 2020.
49. Palmer N. Cancer Survivors in Rural Areas Forgo Health Care Because of Cost. Cancer Epidemiology, Biomarkers and Prevention Oct 2013.
50. Hudis C. The State of Cancer care in America 2014, ASCO Briefing. Available at: http://www.asco.org/practice-reseach/cancer-care-america. Accessed January 27, 2020.
51. Nathan H, Thumma J, Norton E, et al. Strategies for reducing population surgical costs in medicare: local referrals to low-cost hospitals. Ann Surg 2018;267(No. 5):878–85.
52. Bolwell B. Time to treat in cancer patients. Cleveland (OH): Cleveland Clinic Taussig Cancer Center Cancer Advances; 2017.
53. Khorana A, Tullio K, Elson P, et al. Increase in time to initiating cancer therapy and association with worsened survival in curative settings: A US analysis of common solid tumors. J Clin Oncol 2017;35(15 Suppl):16–7.
54. Smith E, Ziogas A, Anton-Culver H. Delay in surgical treatment and survival after breast cancer diagnosis in young women by race/ethnicity. JAMA Surg 2013;148(No. 6):516–23.
55. Bilimoria K, Ko C, Tomlinson J, et al. Wait Times for Cancer Surgery in the US: trends and predictors of delays. Ann Surg 2011;253(4):779–85.
56. Elit L. Wait times from diagnosis to treatment in cancer. J Gynecol Oncol 2015;26(No. 4):246–8.
57. Satiani B, Etzioni D, Williams T. Trends in the General Surgery Workforce. Semin Colon Rectal Surg 2013;24(4):180–6.
58. Ellison E, Pawlik T, Way D, et al. Ten-year reassessment of the shortage of general surgeons: increases in graduation numbers of general surgery residents are insufficient to meet future demand for general surgeons. Surgery 2018;164(Issue 4):726–32.
59. Ellison E, Pawlick T, Way D, et al. The impact of the aging population and incidence of cancer on future projections of general surgical workforce needs. Surgery 2018;163:553–9.
60. Casey M, Barton B, Hung P, et al. Critical access hospital year 7 hospital compare participation and quality measure results. Flex Monitoring Team Briefing

Paper #30, August 2012 30. Available at: http://www.flexmonitoring.org/documents/BriefingPaper30_HospitalCompare.pdf. Accessed January 27, 2020.
61. Gadzinski T, Dimick J, Ye Z, et al. Utilization and outcomes of inpatient surgical care at critical access hospitals in the US. JAMA Surg 2013;148(7):589–96.
62. Ibrahim A, Hughes T, Thumma J, et al. Association of hospital critical access status with surgical outcomes and expenditures among medicare beneficiaries. JAMA 2016;315(No. 19):2095–103.
63. Ibriham A, Regenbogen S, Thumma J, et al. Emergency surgery for medicare beneficiaries admitted to critical access hospitals. Ann Surg 2018;267(3):473–7.
64. Natafgi N, Baloh J, Weigel P, et al. Surgical patient safety outcomes in critical access hospitals: how do they compare? J Rural Health 2017;33(2):117–26.
65. Charlton M. Population-Based Assessment of Patient Rurality, Commission on Cancer Accreditation Status of Cancer Treatment Facility and Quality of Care. 2019 American College of Surgeons Quality and Safety Conference Presentation. Washington, DC, July 19-22, 2019.
66. Winckworth-Prejsner K, lentz L, Nardi E, et al. Value tools for patients in cancer care. J Natl Compr Cancer Netw 2017;15(No. 7):872–7.
67. American College of Surgeons Surgical Risk Calculator. Available at: riskcalculator.facs.org. Accessed January 27, 2020.

Perioperative Support in the Rural Surgery World

Riann Robbins, MD[a], Randall Zuckerman, MD[b,*]

KEYWORDS

- Rural surgery • Preoperative care • Critical access hospital

KEY POINTS

- Surgery in rural environments provides a unique set of challenges.
- The safety and quality of surgery in rural areas should not differ from urban areas.
- Standardization of processes will help achieve these goals.

INTRODUCTION

Perioperative support in a rural surgical environment encompasses unique challenges but ultimately should not substantially differ from those in resource-rich, urban hospitals. Perioperative support can be divided into 5 different phases of care, each with their own resource needs and challenges. These phases include (1) preoperative phase, (2) immediate preoperative phase, (3) intraoperative phase, (4) postoperative phase, and (5) postdischarge phase.

PREOPERATIVE PHASE OUTLINE

The preoperative phase is dedicated to the initial evaluation and diagnosis of the surgical patient before dedicated surgical planning. There are 2 distinct locations where this evaluation occurs: (1) within an outpatient clinic or (2) hospital system, such as within the emergency department or hospital ward. Regardless of the location of the surgical evaluation, the same general principles apply.

Initial outpatient evaluation of preoperative surgical patients relies on a dedicated referral system either from referring providers or direct marketing to the public about available surgical services provided to the community. Unlike urban areas, many patients who seek medical care within a rural environment must travel long distances for medical evaluation contributing to the complexity of providing care to this unique

[a] Department of Surgery, University of Utah, 30 North 1900 East, Salt Lake City, UT 84132, USA; [b] Department of Surgery, Kalispell Regional Medical Center, Kalispell Regional Healthcare, 1333 Surgical Services Drive, Kalispell, MT 59901, USA
* Corresponding author.
E-mail address: RZUCKERMAN@KRMC.ORG

Surg Clin N Am 100 (2020) 893–900
https://doi.org/10.1016/j.suc.2020.06.008

patient population. Therefore, rural surgeons should place a heightened emphasis on developing a comprehensive referral system with other facilities and primary care providers within their region to best provide comprehensive care to a rural population.

Clinical evaluation in the perioperative setting includes a standard basic evaluation by the surgeon which incorporates a full medical history of the patient, a thorough physical examination, and dedicated education about the surgical disease process at hand. As part of this comprehensive evaluation, surgeons should have ready access to basic laboratory and radiologic services.

Minimum necessary radiographic studies including radiography, computed tomography (CT), ultrasound, mammography, MRI, nuclear medicine (NM), and fluoroscopy (FL). Of these, radiography, CT, and ultrasound should be readily available at all times of day to assist with evaluation of urgent problems. Additional specialized radiologic services available to the population within a reasonable time frame should include MRI, mammography, NM, and FL. These specialized radiographic tests may be available by mobile imaging centers if not available on a permanent basis.

Further necessary resources to aid in the preoperative evaluations of surgical patients include laboratory studies. A standard medical laboratory must be available at all times within the surgical facility to collect and process standard analysis of blood, urine, and other bodily fluids; coagulation studies; and blood gas analysis, as well as microbiology studies. Specialized laboratory studies may not be readily processed on site; in this instance, the rural facility should have contractual relationships with outside laboratories to provide a comprehensive workup of rare or unique laboratory studies.

Similar to metropolitan centers, rural populations need access to emergent care such as through an emergency department or urgent care clinic to assist with the evaluation and management of urgent and emergent surgical consults. Emergency department or urgent care personnel must be able to provide assistance in rapid stabilization of critically ill surgical patients including intubation, resuscitation, and administration of Advance Trauma Life Support (ATLS). Surgical providers should be available to provide additional resuscitation efforts, including tube thoracostomy, central access, or Focused Assessment with Ultrasound in Trauma (FAST examination), as dictated by the patient's needs. Rural surgeons must have a dedicated call system for their rural facilities to assist with consultation of urgent and emergent surgical consults.

Perioperative evaluation includes optimization of the patient's comorbid health conditions traditionally with an emphasis on cardiopulmonary disease processes. The American College of Surgeons has developed a preoperative optimization checklist as part of their Strong for Surgery program.[1,2] This unique program focuses on preoperative modifiable risks to optimize patient's health status before elective surgery. Specific areas addressed include nutrition, glycemic control, medication management, smoking cessation, postoperative pain management, delirium, prehabilitation, and patient directives. Strong for Surgery checklists are used to screen patients for risk factors that may lead to surgical complications thereby identifying specific presurgical interventions aimed to improve surgical outcomes. Rural surgery centers should consider including the Strong for Surgery program as a key component of their perioperative evaluation, as described in **Box 1**.

Medical optimization may delay elective surgery if patients require further evaluation and management by primary care providers. Collaborative efforts with anesthesia and pharmacy colleagues may be required to identify additional diagnostic examination and/or changes to the patient's medication before surgery. Rural hospital systems should invest in the development of specific perioperative evaluation clinics aimed at evaluation and optimization of a patient's comorbid conditions before elective surgeries.

Box 1
Strong for surgery components

Nutrition

Glycemic control

Medication management

Smoking cessation

Postoperative pain management

Delirium prevention

Prehabilitation

Patient directives

IMMEDIATE PREOPERATIVE PHASE

The immediate preoperative phase process should mirror that at any larger hospital. Often the same staff will be responsible for both preoperative and postoperative care. Infection prevention protocols should follow published guidelines. Enhanced recoveries after surgery (ERAS) algorithms are easily adaptable to the rural environment.

Special attention must be paid when there is in anticipation of blood products being needed. Rural hospitals have blood banks of varying capability and par levels. If excessive or unusual blood products are going to be needed or anticipated, advance planning is required.

INTRAOPERATIVE PHASE

The intraoperative phase includes procuring a dedicated operative room (OR) or procedural suite with the necessary equipment, resources, perioperative support staff, and surgical team. Rural surgeons face unique obstacles in the intraoperative phase given limitations of smaller medical centers compared with their urban counterparts.

Ideally, a dedicated operating room and/or procedure suite would be available and staffed 24 hours a day, 7 days a week, 365 days a year for any emergent surgical or interventional procedures performed at the facility. The minimum staff required to form a complete surgical team include a preoperative nurse, OR circulating nurse, OR scrub technician, staff surgeon, anesthesia provider, and post anesthesia care unit (PACU) nurse. In rural hospitals, some of these roles may be performed by the same person. The dedicated surgical team must be available on call to provide timely care for any emergent/urgent surgical needs. Response times vary by institution. If operative staff are not available continuously, a documented contingency plan must be in place to cover any gaps in coverage of the surgical team to ensure consistent surgical coverage at the rural facility. Often this contingency plan involves coordinating with hospital administration to hire locums staff to cover call shifts or establishment of concrete transfer protocols with dedicated referral sites with immediately available surgical care.

There are multiple models to provide seamless surgical care. Rural hospitals are a heterogeneous group with some providing operative services at all times. Many others will not be able to provide operative services continuously, and often will transfer patients to a nearby facility. For this to work well, there needs to be good communication and relationships between surgeons at the rural facility and the referral hospital. This allows a bidirectional relationship that benefits patients regarding follow-up and long-term care.

At least 1 qualified surgeon must be actively practicing at the facility. This surgeon should be appropriately credentialed, board-certified or board-eligible, with the necessary skills to perform procedures within a defined scope of practice as outlined by the hospital. If a staff surgeon is not available on call at the hospital, the hospital may support their surgical program with the recruitment of locum tenens surgeons or transfer arrangements.

Anesthesia services must also be available at the facility. These services can be performed by a qualified, credentialed board-certified or board-eligible anesthesia physician or a certified nurse anesthetist.

In addition to specialized personnel necessary for surgery, the hospital requires a specific location to perform surgeries. The operating room and/or procedure suite is a highly specialized location that requires dedicated equipment to function optimally. Each operating room will require different equipment based on the type of procedure being performed and can be customized based on surgeon and facility preferences.

However, a minimum standard of necessary equipment for an operating room and/or procedural suite is as follows:

- Utility column
- Surgical or examination lights
- Surgical table and associated accessories:
  - Anesthesia screens
  - Arm and hand surgery tables
  - Arm supports
  - Clamps
  - Drain pans, hoops, and screens
  - Head supports
  - Leg supports
  - Positioners
  - Restraint straps
  - Side extensions
  - Transfer boards
  - Cushions and mattresses
  - Padding (ie, gel padding)
- Patient transfer devices (ie, gurneys)
- Surgical table, mayo stands
- Sterilizing and cleaning equipment
- Laparotomy equipment
- Laparoscopy equipment
- Digital integration system
- Digital screens
- Self-retaining retractor system
- Gastrointestinal stapling systems
- Endoscopy instruments
- Personal protective equipment
  - Gloves, masks, gowns, shoe covers, bouffant, and so forth

POSTOPERATIVE PHASE

The postoperative phase encompasses the natural transition from the operative/procedural suite into a dedicated area capable of postoperative monitoring and disposition.

All patients who have received general, regional, or monitored anesthesia require transfer to either a dedicated PACU or equivalent area where the patient is observed by personnel trained to recognize and manage immediate postoperative complications Policies and procedure outlined by the hospital's Department of Anesthesia generally govern the medical care of the patients during this time. Patients transported from the OR to the PACU or similar area should be accompanied by a member of the anesthesia team who is capable of continued evaluation and treatment of the patient during transport. On PACU arrival, the patient's condition will be reevaluated by dedicated PACU nursing staff and transition of care will take place from the member of the anesthesia team to the PACU nurse. Protocols for ongoing reevaluation, including vital sign checks and clinical examination, should be clearly established. A predetermined checklist of objective measures should dictate when the patient is eligible for transfer out of the PACU to the next phase of care.[3] Standard discharge criteria are described in **Box 2**.

PACU disposition varies depending on preoperative expectation, intraoperative assessment, and patient response to anesthesia. Determination of proper disposition involves close collaboration between nursing staff and surgeon with input from the anesthesia team. Similar to immediate personnel required to maintain a functional OR staff, the PACU must be equipped and appropriately staffed 24 hours a day, 7 days a week, 365 days a year, or whenever operative services are provided.

Patients who are ineligible to discharge home from the PACU after surgery may require a brief period of convalescence within the hospital until they are safe to discharge. The hospital must designate an area for inpatient management of surgical patients equipped with dedicated staff specifically trained in the management of surgical patients. This involves a multidisciplinary team of professionals, including nursing staff, and physical, occupational, respiratory, and speech therapy, as well as wound care and nutritional experts. Preferably, members from each ancillary discipline should meet at regular intervals with the surgeon to discuss optimal hospital disposition of patients who remain in house. The focus of these meetings should regularly reassess the readiness of disposition of the patient from the hospitalization. The likely disposition of patients after their initial period of convalescence includes discharge to home, a skilled nursing facility, or transfer to inpatient rehabilitation. This decision is generally

Box 2
Standard patient discharge criteria

- Patent airway and respiratory function
- Stable vital signs
- Appropriate perfusion
- Appropriate or baseline mental status
- Normothermia
- Adequate pain control
- Patent intravenous vascular access
- Absence of bladder distention and adequate urine output if applicable
- Intact and patent surgically placed tubes, drains, or other catheters
- Lack of surgical bleeding or wound drainage
- Intact surgical dressings

guided by the collective assessment of providers and ancillary services and implemented by a social worker or case manager in coordination with the surgical provider.

Geographic and socioeconomic pressures unique to a rural environment complicate discharge planning. Patients may not have access to outpatient therapies in smaller communities and, therefore, longer length of admission may be required.

Patient status and needs may change throughout their postoperative care. Postoperative management therefore involves ongoing clinical evaluation, which may drive the need for higher level of care including intensive care management. Rural hospitals may benefit from providing short-term intensive care to postsurgical patients, thereby reducing costly transfers to outside facilities. Contingency plans for emergent transfer must include established protocols for transfer to larger regional medical centers if the needs of the patient exceed the resources available at the rural hospital. The ability to keep an intubated or critically ill patient at a rural facility varies tremendously. Careful preoperative thought and planning are required to avoid the situation if intensive care resources are not locally available.

Ancillary support services available for the management of inpatient surgical patients include access to radiologic, laboratory, and pharmacy services similar to the outpatient setting. Radiologic capabilities immediately available at all times should include radiography, CT, and ultrasound.

Discharge planning ideally starts in the preoperative phase, but as patients near the completion of their hospital course, health care teams prepare for the transition of patient care beyond the hospital environment. Just as the transition from the PACU to the next phase of care is protocolized, so too should the transition between the hospital back to the community or the next phase of the patient's care. The discharge summary is one of the most important communication records for this pivotal transition, and standardization of included information can help enhance this critical period of the perioperative environment, especially for a rural hospital system, as evidenced in **Box 3**.[4]

POSTDISCHARGE PHASE

The postdischarge phase of perioperative support focuses on the development of protocols and pathways for long-term follow-up and communication between providers after the patient has been discharged from the hospital.

Patients require close follow-up with the operating surgeon within an appropriate time frame. Typically this follow-up occurs 1 to 2 weeks after discharge to assessment of postoperative recovery, development of any surgical complications, and follow up on any necessary imaging or laboratory studies. Data also suggest early postoperative visits with primary care physicians reduce 30-day hospital readmissions.[5] Therefore, close communication between the surgeon, primary care physician, and other specialist should be standard to provide comprehensive postsurgical care.

Rural hospital systems need an associated emergency room (ER) capable of assessing patients for possible readmission. The ER must have the capability to obtain appropriate imaging and laboratory studies to diagnose postsurgical complications. Open lines of communication between ER providers and facility surgeons are vital to the management of postoperative complications.

QUALITY IMPROVEMENT INITIATIVES AND TOOLS

Many improvement initiatives and tools are available to help rural facilities and surgeons ensure quality care is provided to their community. Rural hospitals should have systems in place to collect surgical outcome data and provide surveillance

Box 3
Minimum information included on a standard discharge summary

Principal diagnosis

Operation procedure type, date, primary surgeon

Operative/perioperative complications

Active medical problems managed

Changes to medication, with rationale and plan for represcribing and deprescribing

Anticipated postdischarge course, including specific information regarding wound care, mobilization advice, driving and nutrition

Discussions of anticipated escalation of care or need for readmission

Recent blood results and requests for ongoing monitoring after discharge

Safety-netting, including who to contact for more information

both for the facility as well as individual surgeons to assist with the identification of potential quality and safety issues. Two nationally recognized programs include the American College of Surgeons National Surgical Quality Improvement Program (ACS NSQIP)[6] and the ACS Surgeon-Specific Registry (ACS SSR).[7]

The ACS NSQIP is a nationally validated, risk-adjusted, outcomes-based program that aims to measure and improve the quality of surgical care within hospitals. The goal of the ACS NSQIP program is to help enrolled hospital systems improve their surgical care through the use of risk-adjusted clinical data. The program captures and reports 30-day morbidity and mortality outcomes for all major inpatient and outpatient surgical procedures to help hospitals identify areas unique to their hospital that can be targeted for improvement. Rural hospital systems are strongly encouraged to consider enrollment in this national program and may obtain more information on the ACS Web site: www.FACS.org. An additional feature of the ACS NSQIP program nationally is an online risk calculator that can be used by any surgeon regardless of facility participation in the ACS NSQIP program to assist with objective calculation of the surgical patient's risk assessment perioperatively. This online risk calculator can be found at https://riskcalculator.facs.org/RiskCalculator/.

The ACS SSR is an online quality improvement tool and database that allows individual surgeons to track their outcomes and cases. This service is provided free of charge to members of the ACS or for a small fee for nonmembers. Benefits of the program allow for surgeon-specific tracking of cases and outcomes, data analysis and reporting, and ability to meet regulatory requirements of the American Board of Surgeons and Centers for Medicare and Medicaid Services Merit-based Incentive Payment System. Information on enrollment into the program may also be obtained at www.FACS.org.

In addition, the newly launched Rural Surgery Standards Program provides a comprehensive evaluation of surgical capabilities and standards across rural hospitals. This program is still in a pilot phase, but certainly has the promise of ensuring that surgery in the rural environment is held to a consistent and high standard across the country.

SUMMARY

Perioperative surgical standards are consistent between a rural and urban medical environment; however, implementation of those standards can be more challenging in a rural setting. Unique circumstances to consider in establishing perioperative support systems in a rural environment include consideration of reduced medical resources, such as personnel, limited access to ancillary services, and large geographic distances of patient travel and referral networks. Despite these unique challenges to overcome, thoughtful design of the perioperative surgical support system can be implemented successfully in a rural surgical environment.

DISCLOSURE

The authors have nothing to disclose.

REFERENCES

1. American College of Surgeons. Strong For Surgery. Available at: https://www.facs.org/quality-programs/strong-for-surgery. Accessed March 20, 2020.
2. Committee on Standards and Practice Parameters. Standards for Postanesthesia Care. 2019. Available at: https://www.asahq.org/standards-and-guidelines/standards-for-postanesthesia-care. Accessed May 11, 2020.
3. Glick D, Holt N, Nussmeier N. Overview of post-anesthetic care for adult patients [Internet]. UpToDate. 2020. Available at: https://www.uptodate.com/contents/overview-of-post-anesthetic-care-for-adult-patients#H2860377297. Accessed May 14, 2020.
4. Bougeard AM, Watkins B. Transitions of care in the perioperative period – A review. Clin Med J R Coll Physicians London 2019;19(6):446–9.
5. Brooke BS, Goodney PP, Kraiss LW, et al. Readmission destination and risk of mortality after major surgery: an observational cohort study. Lancet 2015;386(9996):884–95.
6. American College of Surgeons. ACS National Surgical Quality Improvement Program [Internet]. Available at: https://www.facs.org/quality-programs/acs-nsqip. Accessed May 11, 2020.
7. American College of Surgeons. Surgeon Specific Registry [Internet]. Available at: https://www.facs.org/quality-programs/ssr. Accessed May 11, 2020.

Rural Surgical Quality

Policy and Practice

Amy L. Halverson, MD, MHPE

KEYWORDS

• Rural surgery • Quality improvement • Risk-adjustment • Quality collaborative • Quality measures • Patient selection • Cancer outcomes

KEY POINTS

- Rural hospitals often have limited resources and face challenges in caring for patients and communities with sociodemographic and geographic barriers to care. As such, defining quality in the rural context requires consideration of various factors in identifying rural-relevant metrics, analyzing outcomes, and targeting interventions for quality improvement.
- Studies evaluating quality surgical care in rural areas incorporate data at the national, regional and institutional levels. National studies using risk-adjusted administrative data show that surgical care in rural communities is comparable to care in urban centers. Regional studies include outcomes for specific diseases including various cancers. Studies have also examined specific procedures such as colonoscopy.
- Rural hospitals, of which many are critical access hospitals, must perform quality improvement with limited financial resources and personnel who play several roles within the hospital. Furthermore, a small quality improvement team must address quality improvement beyond the scope of surgical care. These hospitals can leverage expertise in project implementation and data analysis by participating in state and regional quality collaboratives.

INTRODUCTION

Rural hospitals often have limited resources and face challenges in caring for patients and communities with sociodemographic and geographic barriers to care. As such, defining quality in the rural context requires consideration of various factors in identifying rural-relevant metrics, analyzing outcomes, and targeting interventions for quality improvement. Barriers to measuring quality performance include relatively low volumes and limited resources for quality improvement.

PATIENT FACTORS AND COMMUNITY FACTORS

Contextualization in quality improvement accounts for patient and community characteristics, such as health-related behavior, access to health care services, and

Northwestern University Feinberg School of Medicine, 676 North Street Clair, Suite 650, Chicago, IL 60611, USA
E-mail address: amy.halverson@nm.org

Surg Clin N Am 100 (2020) 901–908
https://doi.org/10.1016/j.suc.2020.07.001 surgical.theclinics.com

environmental exposures. Understanding how patient and sociodemographic factors affect health outcomes allows for a more accurate comparison of rural care against other settings and a more meaningful interpretation of quality data. Rural communities in the United States generally are disadvantaged relative to urban or suburban areas, particularly with respect to economics, education, health status, and access to the health care delivery system. Individuals in these communities are more likely to be older, engage in poor health behaviors such as smoking, and have higher mortality rates for cardiovascular disease and cancer. Rural residents also have lower income, are less likely to have health insurance, and have lower educational attainment.[1–3] They also are more likely to experience difficulties accessing primary, emergency, dental, and mental health care.[4,5]

Hennin-Smith and colleagues[6] attempted to elucidate which factors to consider for risk adjustment in quality analysis in the rural setting. They compiled patient and community factors and compared outcomes based on rurality. They evaluated 6 quality of care measures (satisfaction with care, blood pressure checked, cholesterol checked, flu shot receipt, change in health status, and all-cause annual readmission) from the Medicare Current Beneficiary Survey Access to Care module, which contained questions about beneficiaries' experiences with care and sociodemographic information. County-level data came from the 2012 County Health Rankings (CHR), a database developed at the University of Wisconsin Population Health Institute, which includes statistics on health and sociodemographic information. Individual factors included minutes it takes for patients to get to their usual provider ($<$30 minutes vs $\geq$30 minutes), level of education, self-rated health status, living arrangement/marital status (married and living with a spouse, living alone, or living with someone else), sex, age, and race/ethnicity. County-level characteristics included the percentage of residents age 65 or older, access to a grocery store (access to healthy foods), percentage of adults who are obese, county unemployment rate, percentage of children in poverty, percentage of adults who report that they have no social or emotional support, and percentage of adults without a high school degree. The investigators found that patients from rural areas were more likely to self-classify as white, non-Hispanic. The rural patients had higher rates of obesity, higher unemployment, higher rates of children in poverty, lower self-reported levels of health, lower social/emotional support, and fewer primary care physicians. Rural residents had similar unadjusted average scores for each quality measure. With risk adjustment, however, rural patients were less likely to have cholesterol screening. A key finding of this study was that even when adjusting for community and individual characteristics, rurality still was associated with differences in quality of care.[6]

In evaluating urban and rural health disparities, Long and colleagues[7] evaluated factors contributing to premature mortality, defined as death before age 75, in rural populations. Using Area Health Resources Files from the US Health Resources and Service Administration and CHR data to model mortality with and without urban-rural coding, the investigators found that mortality rates were explained primarily by socioeconomic variables. The investigators concluded that addressing the social determinants of health is likely to be more effective than targeting the health care system and that more research is needed to understand better how culture mitigates the effect of socioeconomic variables on health outcomes.[7] DeJager and colleagues[8] evaluated the impact of income on outcomes after emergency general surgery procedures. Using data from the Nationwide Inpatient Sample, they compared risk-adjusted postoperative outcomes based on income and rural status. The investigators found that low income was associated with worse outcomes in urban but not rural settings.

Casey and colleagues[9] reported the results of an expert panel convened to identify quality measures relevant for critical access hospitals (CAHs). The group developed a framework for measures that account for low patient volume, internal usefulness for quality improvement, and external usefulness of quality reporting and payment. The panel evaluated existing Centers for Medicare & Medicaid Services inpatient and outpatient quality reporting and electronic health record meaningful use measures as well as the Joint Commission and National Quality Forum (NQF)–endorsed measures. Surgical care measures included perioperative antibiotic prophylaxis and venous thromboembolism prophylaxis, urinary catheter removal on postoperative day 1, and perioperative temperature control. These measures apply to a wide range of surgical procedures. The panel recommended that future surgical quality measures include a surgical checklist measure and high-volume outpatient procedures, such as endoscopy and colonoscopy.[9]

In 2014, the NQF convened an expert panel to address sociodemographic factors. The panel recognized that social and economic factors in addition to a patient's health status and the quality of health care treatments affect patient outcomes. The panel established guiding principles for rural quality measures that include utilizing metrics that are feasible for data collection by rural providers, that is, measures that rely on readily available data or data that are feasible to collect. The measures should be broadly applicable to compensate for low volumes in rural hospitals and useful for internal quality improvement efforts. The panel recommended that future assessments of care quality include risk adjustment for community-level variables, including travel distance to provider, social support, and socioeconomic factors.[10]

In 2018, the NQF[11] further recognized that there are social and economic factors related specifically to care in rural communities that are important to consider when assessing quality. The organization proposed several quality measures that were relevant to rural practice, meaningful even with low case volumes, and risk adjusted for rural sociodemographic factors (**Box 1**). Considerations for relevant factors included access to care, especially to specialists; health literacy; and affordability.[11] Although

Box 1
Surgery-relevant quality measures for rural hospitals

Catheter-associated urinary tract infection

HCAHPS

Falls with injury

Emergency transfer communication measure

Venous thromboembolism prophylaxis

Cesarean birth

Alcohol use screening

Inpatient hospital-onset *Clostridium difficile* infection outcome measure

Hospital-wide, all-cause unplanned readmission

Data from National Quality Forum. Performance measurement for rural low-volume providers: final report by the NQF Rural Health Committee September 14, 2015. Available at: http://www.qualityforum.org/Publications/2015/09/Rural_Health_Final_Report.aspx.

there was a consensus that sociodemographic factors should be calculated into risk-adjusted outcomes, how best to incorporate these factors warrants further study.

SURGICAL QUALITY

Despite the challenges outlined previously, data from several studies comparing risk-adjusted outcomes of surgical care in rural hospitals or CAHs to urban hospitals show that rural hospitals provide care that is comparable to care at larger, urban hospitals. Gadzinski and coauthors[12] analyzed data from the American Hospital Administration and the National Inpatient Sample to compare mortality, length of stay, and cost at CAHs and prospective payment system (PPS) hospitals with fewer than 50 beds. The investigators found that compared with patients in the PPS hospitals, CAH patients were slightly younger (55 years old vs 57 years old, respectively) and had fewer comorbid conditions (3.1 vs 3.7, respectively). Operative mortality was similar in patients for 7 of the most commonly performed procedures, which included appendectomy, cholecystectomy, colectomy, cesarean section, hysterectomy, and knee replacement. One exception was an increase in mortality after hip fracture repair or replacement among Medicare recipients treated at CAHs (adjusted odds ratio = 1.37; 95% CI, 1.01 to 1.87). The investigators opined that increased morality from hip fracture repair might reflect the urgent treatment of older patients with more comorbidities. An additional finding was that despite shorter lengths of stay ($P<.001$ for 4 procedures), costs at CAHs were higher ($P<.001$) for all 8 procedures.[12] Natafgi and coauthors[13] utilized the Healthcare Cost and utilization Project State Inpatient Databases, sponsored by the Agency for Healthcare Research and Quality, and used the American Hospital Association data to identify CAHs They evaluate provider-level patient safety indicators, including death, postoperative hemorrhage and hematoma, postoperative respiratory failure, perioperative pulmonary embolism or venous thromboembolism, postoperative sepsis, or wound dehiscence. They also found similar rates of complications in CAHs compared with other small (fewer than 50 beds) non-CAH hospitals. Patients at CAHs were slightly younger and had fewer comorbidities. After adjusting for patient and hospital characteristics, the investigators found that CAHs' performance was the same or better than that of the small community hospitals for all indicators. The investigators opined that increased quality might be related to improved reimbursement, increased complexity of cases at other hospitals, and a closer relationship with general surgeons and their patients in the rural setting.

Ibrahim and coauthors[14] add more evidence that CAHs provide high-quality and cost-effective care. The investigators conducted a retrospective review of more than 1 million Medicare beneficiary admissions for 1 of 4 common surgical procedures, including appendectomy, cholecystectomy, colectomy, and hernia repair. The investigators found that CAHs had mortality and morbidity rates that were comparable to non-CAHs.[14] CAHs had significantly lower rates of serious complications (6.4% vs 13.9%, respectively; OR 0.35; 95% CI, 0.32–0.39; $P<.001$). Furthermore, Medicare expenditures adjusted for patient factors and procedure type were lower at CAHs than at non-CAHs . ($14,450 vs $15,845, respectively; $P<.001$). In a subsequent study, Ibrahim and colleagues[15] utilized the Medicare Provider Analysis and Review database to compare outcomes after emergency colectomy procedures CAHs and non-CAHs. Complications included pulmonary failure, pneumonia, myocardial infarction, deep venous thrombosis, acute renal failure, surgical site infection, and gastrointestinal bleeding. The investigators found that compared with patients treated at non-CAHs, patients undergoing surgery at CAHs were less likely to have multiple comorbid diseases (percentage of patients with 2 or more comorbid conditions, 67.5% vs 75.9%, respectively; $P<.01$). They also found that mortality was lower at CAHs. In comparing 30-day risk-adjusted outcomes, the investigators found that CAHs also had lower rates of serious complications but higher rates of reoperation and readmission. Of patients treated at CAHs, 7.3% required to transfer to another acute hospital facility compared with only 1.2% of patients requiring a transfer at non-CAHs. All of the studies, described previously, utilized administrative databases to compare outcomes in CAHs and non-CAHs using risk adjustment for patient factors. Studies utilizing administrative data provide broad information about the collective performance of rural hospitals, which may be useful for health care policy. These studies do not provide actionable guidance to individual hospitals or providers.

Gadzinski and colleagues[12] and Ibrahim and colleagues[14] showed fewer patient comorbidities in the CAH cohorts. One explanation might be that rural providers transferred more complex patients to larger hospitals. Two recent studies examined transfer patterns in rural hospitals. Windorski and colleagues[16] compared outcomes of 394 patients treated initially at a level I trauma center versus 1084 patients stabilized at a CAH and then transferred to a level I trauma center in Kansas. The investigators found that the patients transferred from the CAH were older (52.4 years vs 42.2 years, respectively) but did not assess other comorbidities. After controlling for injury severity score, age, Glasgow Comas Scale, and shock, the odds of mortality did not differ between CAH transfer patients and patients transported directly to a level I facility (odds ratio 0.70; $P = .20$). In a second study, Misercola and colleagues,[17] compared nontrauma patients requiring acute general surgical care transferred to a regional center in Maine to patients who presented to the regional center emergency department. The 161 transferred patients (TPs) were older (61.2 years vs 54.7 years, respectively; $P<.001$), had more comorbidities (Charlson Comorbidity Index 4 vs 3.1, respectively; $P<.001$), and required more resources than 611 local patients (LPs) (length of stay 8.2 vs 3.4 days, respectively [$P<.001$]; intensive care unit admission 24% vs 6% of patients, respectively [$P<.001$]). Admission diagnoses were similar, with pancreaticobiliary (TPs 29% vs LPs 30%) and small bowel (TPs 25% vs LPs 23%,) complaints most common. The most common intervention was laparoscopic cholecystectomy for both (29% vs 25%, respectively). Subspecialty interventions were similar (interventional radiology and advanced endoscopy) for TPs, 10%, and LPs, 8%. TPs were more likely not to require a procedure (31% vs 23%, respectively). Insurance providers differed between groups, particularly for Medicare (55% vs 34%, respectively) and privately insured (26% vs 45%, respectively) patients. This study supports the idea that more complex patients are transferred even for basic general surgical care.

Colonoscopy is one of the most common procedures performed by general surgeons. Due to the paucity of gastroenterologists, general surgeons and, increasingly, family practitioners, perform the majority of colonoscopies in rural communities.[18] Holub and colleagues[19] compared colonoscopy performance metrics from rural practitioners in the state of Oregon to benchmarks from nonrural providers. The investigators used data obtained with the use of a commercial endoscopic reporting software application. The investigators compared metrics based on national quality guidelines that included cecal photo documentation rate, withdrawal time, and adenoma detection rate. The colonoscopies in the Oregon rural practices were performed by surgeons (18%) and primary care physicians (69%) in contrast to 18% performed by non-gastroenterologists in nonrural practices. The cecal intubation rate was lower for rural providers (87.4% vs 90.9%, respectively; $P = .002$) and did not meet the recommended goal of 95%. The polyp detection rate was similar (rural, 39%, vs nonrural, 40.3%; $P = .217$).

CANCER CARE

In addition to postoperative outcome measures, several studies have reported outcomes related to specific disease processes. For example, there are several studies that have looked at and evaluated disparities in rural and urban oncologic outcomes. Chow and colleagues[20] used the California Cancer Registry to compare colon cancer outcomes in the rural communities of California. Even after adjusting for patient factors, stage, tumor characteristics, and treatment modality, the approximately 15% of individuals residing in rural areas had worse cancer-specific survival (hazard ratio 1.038; 95% CI, 1.007–1.071; *P* = .016). Rural residents were diagnosed at later stages, were less likely to have had adequate lymphadenectomy, and had a lower likelihood of receiving chemotherapy for stage III disease.[20]

A more recent study compared oncology outcomes in urban and rural areas of Utah, a state that is unique in it low rates of smoking, alcohol consumption, obesity, and younger population. The investigators used the Surveillance, Epidemiology, and End Results Program database and used county-level variables, including education (percentage of at least bachelor's degree and poverty rate, percentage of current smokers, obesity, and pap smear and mammography rates). The investigators found that cancer patients living in rural counties had less education, had lower income, were less likely to have insurance, and had higher rates of smoking and obesity. Both pap smears and mammography were less likely in rural counties. The overall cancer incidence rate was lower in rural areas. In particular, the incidence and survival rates of breast and prostate were lower in the rural counties. In contrast, colon and lung cancers had higher incidence rates in rural counties and similar survival compared with metropolitan counties. Rural residents were less likely to undergo surgery or radiation treatment. For all cancers combined, rural residents had 5.2% lower 5-year relative survival.[21]

STATE COLLABORATIVES

Data from national and statewide administrative databases inform national policy and increase our understanding of what factors that affect patient outcomes. Administrative data has limited utility for driving quality improvement at the institutional level. Much of the published literature on quality improvement efforts in rural hospitals applies to initiatives that are not surgery-specific. For example, there have been several projects aimed at reducing readmissions at rural hospitals. In Minnesota, several organizations, including the Minnesota Hospital Association and Stratis Health, an education and quality improvement consortium, have developed a statewide program to reduce hospital readmissions by improving communication during discharge and transitions of care. Participating hospitals receive support through coaching, technical support, and quarterly reports of readmission data. This effort included 38 CAHs, which collectively realized a mean decrease of 0.34 in observed/expected readmissions.[22]

Similar to the Minnesota collaborative, many states have instituted statewide collaboratives that serve to support hospitals in quality improvement by providing education and mentoring to physicians, nurses, and quality improvement professionals as well as support with abstracted data collection, risk stratification, data analysis, and longitudinal benchmark data.[23] In some states, collaboratives provided start-up stipends and funding for pilot grants. Collaboratives may address a single problem or encompass quality improvement across a range of specialties.[24] These collaboratives are useful especially for rural hospitals, which have limited financial and human resources for quality improvement efforts.

SUMMARY

Several national studies have demonstrated that rural hospitals successfully deliver high-quality care. Data at the national, regional, institutional, and individual practitioner levels all contribute to the understanding of surgical outcomes in the rural setting. Quality metrics should be interpreted within the context of the rural community and outcomes analyzed with relevant risk-adjustment for patient factors.

Rural hospitals, of which many are CAHs, must perform quality improvement with limited financial resources and personnel, who play several roles within the hospital. Furthermore, a small quality improvement team must address quality improvement beyond the scope of surgical care. These hospitals can leverage expertise in project implementation and data analysis by participating in state and regional quality collaboratives.

DISCLOSURE

The author has no disclosures.

REFERENCES

1. New census data show differences between urban and rural populations. Available at: https://www.census.gov/newsroom/press-releases/2016/cb16-210.html. Accessed May 10, 2020.
2. Health-Related Behaviors by Urban-Rural County Classification — United States, 2013. Centers for Disease Control and Prevention. Available at: https://www.cdc.gov/mmwr/volumes/66/ss/ss6605a1.htm#T2_down. Accessed May 10, 2020.
3. State fact sheets: United States. 2020. Available at: https://data.ers.usda.gov/reports.aspx?ID=17854. Accessed May 10, 2020.
4. Douthit N, Kiv S, Dwolatzky T, et al. Exposing some important barriers to health care access in the rural USA. Public Health 2015;129:611–20.
5. Meit MK, A, Gilbert, T, Yu, AT, et al. The 2014 Update of the Rural-Urban Chartbook: The North Dakota and NORC Rural health Reform Policy Research Center (RHRPRC); 2014.
6. Henning-Smith C, Kozhimannil K, Casey M, et al. Rural-urban differences in medicare quality outcomes and the impact of risk adjustment. Med Care 2017; 55:823–9.
7. Long AS, Hanlon AL, Pellegrin KL. Socioeconomic variables explain rural disparities in US mortality rates: Implications for rural health research and policy. SSM Popul Health 2018;6:72–4.
8. DeJager E, Chaudhary MA. The Impact fo Income on Emervency General Surgery Outcomes in Urban and Rural Areas. Journal of Surgical Research 2020; 245:629–35.
9. Casey MM, Moscovice I, Klingner J, et al. Rural relevant quality measures for critical access hospitals. J Rural Health 2013;29:159–71.
10. Performance measurement for rural low-volume providers. National Quality Forum Rural Health Committee; 2015.
11. Rural Health Workgroup of the National Quality Forum. A Core Set of Rural-Relevant Measures and Measuring and Improving Access to Care: 2018 Recommendations from the MAP Rural Health Workgroup. 2018.
12. Gadzinski AJ, Dimick JB, Ye Z, et al. Utilization and outcomes of inpatient surgical care at critical access hospitals in the United States. JAMA Surg 2013;148: 589–96.

13. Natafgi N, Baloh J, Weigel P, et al. Surgical patient safety outcomes in critical access hospitals: how do they compare? J Rural Health 2017;33:117–26.
14. Ibrahim AM, Hughes TG, Thumma JR, et al. Association of hospital critical access status with surgical outcomes and expenditures among medicare beneficiaries. JAMA 2016;315:2095–103.
15. Ibrahim AM, Regenbogen SE, Thumma JR, et al. Emergency surgery for medicare beneficiaries admitted to critical access hospitals. Ann Surg 2018;267: 473–7.
16. Windorski J, Reyes J, Helmer SD, et al. Differences in hospital outcomes following traumatic injury for patients experiencing immediate transfer to a level I trauma facility versus resuscitation at a critical access hospital (CAH). Am J Surg 2019;217:643–7.
17. Misercola B, Sihler K, Douglas M, et al. Transfer of acute care surgery patients in a rural state: a concerning trend. J Surg Res 2016;206:168–74.
18. Komaravolu SS, Kim JJ, Singh S, et al. Colonoscopy utilization in rural areas by general surgeons: An analysis of the National Ambulatory Medical Care Survey. Am J Surg 2019;218:281–7.
19. Holub JL, Morris C, Fagnan LJ, et al. Quality of colonoscopy performed in rural practice: experience from the clinical outcomes research initiative and the oregon rural practice-based research network. J Rural Health 2018;34(Suppl 1):s75–83.
20. Chow CJ, Al-Refaie WB, Abraham A, et al. Does patient rurality predict quality colon cancer care?: A population-based study. Dis Colon Rectum 2015;58:415–22.
21. Hashibe M, Kirchhoff AC, Kepka D, et al. Disparities in cancer survival and incidence by metropolitan versus rural residence in Utah. Cancer Med 2018;7: 1490–7.
22. McCoy KA, Bear-Pfaffendof K, Foreman JK, et al. Reducing avoidable hospital readmissions effectively: a statewide campaign. Jt Comm J Qual Patient Saf 2014;40:198–204.
23. Campbell DA Jr, Kubus JJ, Henke PK, et al. The Michigan surgical quality collaborative: a legacy of Shukri Khuri. Am J Surg 2009;198:S49–55.
24. Berian JR, Thomas JM, Minami CA, et al. Evaluation of a novel mentor program to improve surgical care for US hospitals. Int J Qual Health Care 2017;29:234–42.

Advanced Technology and the Rural Surgeon

Robert P. Sticca, MD*, Kayla J. Burchill, MD, Stefan W. Johnson, MD

KEYWORDS

• Rural surgery • Advanced technology • Robotic surgery • Endoscopy
• Telemedicine

KEY POINTS

- Many types of technologic advances have been developed in the past three decades in medicine and surgery.
- Advanced technology has and continues to change surgical practice.
- Barriers to incorporation of new technologies exist in rural surgery.
- Despite barriers many advanced technologies are appropriate for rural surgeons.

INTRODUCTION

The last three decades have seen radical changes in the practice of surgery. Many of these changes have been enabled by the development, adaptation, and implementation of new technologies in surgery. Minimally invasive (initially laparoscopic) surgery is probably the most visible example of advanced technology altering the status quo in surgery. There are many other instances of new and emerging technologies that will continue to change the way that medicine and surgery is practiced in the future. Although these technologic advances can affect all specialties, the surgical specialties are especially influenced by new and emerging technologies because of the technical nature of surgery and its growing dependence on technology to perform increasingly complex surgeries in ways that result in minimal discomfort and disability and provide improved outcomes for patients.

The adoption and use of advanced technology in surgery has presented several challenges in the surgical specialties. These challenges have become increasingly important in the last few decades as technologic applications have been developed and disseminated with increasing speed. Adequate verification of the benefits, safety, and cost-effectiveness of new technologies is difficult to obtain in a timely fashion. For many new devices and procedures, the race to adopt and use them supersedes the

Department of Surgery, University of North Dakota School of Medicine and Health Sciences, Suite E270, 1301 North Columbia Road, Stop 9037, Grand Forks, ND 58202-9037, USA
* Corresponding author.
E-mail address: robert.sticca@und.edu

https://doi.org/10.1016/j.suc.2020.06.003

rational and scientific evaluation of the technology. The haste to adopt new technologies has been influenced by competition within the health care system and pressure applied by commercial vendors, advertising, and perceptions of the lay public. Adequate training, credentialing, and minimal requirements to develop expertise in new technologies continues to be an issue with several major surgical societies developing voluntary guidelines for the adoption of new technologies and procedures.[1–4] The current health care system in the United States has many competing interests, including governmental funding, third-party payors, pharmaceutical and device manufacturers, individual health care systems, physicians, and their patients, all of whom have their own views and interests when new technologies are introduced. The cost of new technologies is expensive and sometimes prohibitive because manufacturers, technology developers, health care consultants, and data managers all must cover research and developmental costs and potential litigation costs for their technologies. Despite the cost of new technology, many hospitals and health care systems have chosen to invest in these technologies seeking improved outcomes, patient satisfaction, and efficiency.

The adoption of new technology in rural hospitals often presents greater challenges because the issues encountered in larger health systems and academic medical centers is magnified and at times become almost insurmountable for smaller rural facilities. Although the implementation and use of new and advanced technologies in small rural hospitals is of benefit to the hospital and patients, it is more difficult because of intrinsic barriers inherent in rural surgery practice. These include the cost of the new technology, training of surgeons and staff, administrative and clinical support, ability to maintain proficiency because of low volume, restrictions on patients and length of stay, and concerns for quality monitoring. Some technologies are better suited for rural practices (eg, telemedicine) and allow for the provision of medical services that would not normally be available in rural locations. Others are better suited for major academic centers where the volumes and referral patterns are conducive to the adoption, usage, and monitoring of new and advanced technologies. Because of the nature of rural communities and hospitals, which in many cases can only support one or two surgeons, the rural surgeon is often the primary force in deciding on and implementing new technologies in rural hospitals and surgical programs.

The topic of new and advanced technologies in medicine and surgery is broad, with many new innovations and technologies in development or existence. A detailed discussion of all new and developing technologies is beyond the scope of this article. Here we discuss some of the advantages, challenges, and limitations in the use of advanced technologies in rural locations. Although the pertinent factors for the implementation and use of advanced technology in rural locations varies depending on the location, hospital, and surgeon, some common conclusions can be drawn that may be applicable to many technologies and locations. We elucidate these with examples in three major areas of technology (operative, endoscopic, and telemedicine), which in our opinion are currently important to rural surgeons. There is an abundance of information for each of these areas that could fill an entire journal or monograph but we summarize them and discuss their relevance and applicability to a rural surgeon's practice.

OPERATIVE TECHNOLOGIES

Robotic Surgery

Use of robotic-assisted platforms has been increasing rapidly in several specialties including urology, gynecology, cardiothoracic surgery, and general surgery. Current evidence suggests that the benefits of robotic surgery when compared with laparoscopic surgery include stabilization of instruments, mechanical advantages over traditional laparoscopy, improved ergonomics for the operating surgeon, and superior visualization incorporating three-dimensional imaging of the operative field.[5] Clinically, however, initial reports on robotic surgery demonstrated that outcomes were equivalent to established laparoscopic techniques, and costs could be up to 25% higher. Despite these concerns, robotic surgery for common surgical procedures has risen dramatically. From 2012 to 2018, colectomy, inguinal hernia repair, and ventral hernia repair saw a 6-, 41-, and 44-fold increase in use (**Fig. 1**).[6]

As robotic technology becomes more commonplace the question arises whether it is appropriate in the rural environment. Regionalization, surgeon recruitment and training, and economics are all factors that play a part in determining whether robotic surgery is appropriate in rural locations.

Regionalization of care is of particular concern to rural hospitals. Common surgical procedures that were once performed regularly in a rural hospital are more often being referred to high-volume centers. Rural hospitals may feel pressure to adopt the technology as surgeries are lost to other hospitals. High-volume centers are also more likely to use robotic approaches. In areas where robotics has become common, regionalization of cancer surgery has occurred. This has been especially true for radical prostatectomy.[7] In recent years, general surgery has been the fastest growing adopter of robotics. As robotic surgery increases in general surgery practices, the effect on rural hospitals without robotic capabilities is devastating. Loss of rural general surgeons can have significant consequences to a rural hospital, financial and clinical. Sixty percent of rural hospitals in North Dakota have stopped providing obstetric care because of loss of a general surgeon, or inability to recruit.[8] Endoscopy and minimally invasive surgery are the cornerstones of any rural surgeon. Screening and diagnostic endoscopy provides an opportunity to identify surgically correctable pathology that, when appropriate, can be performed in the rural setting.[9] If the rural surgeon does not have the best tools to surgically address a problem, the patient may seek care elsewhere. It is a financial loss to the local health care system, not to mention a burden

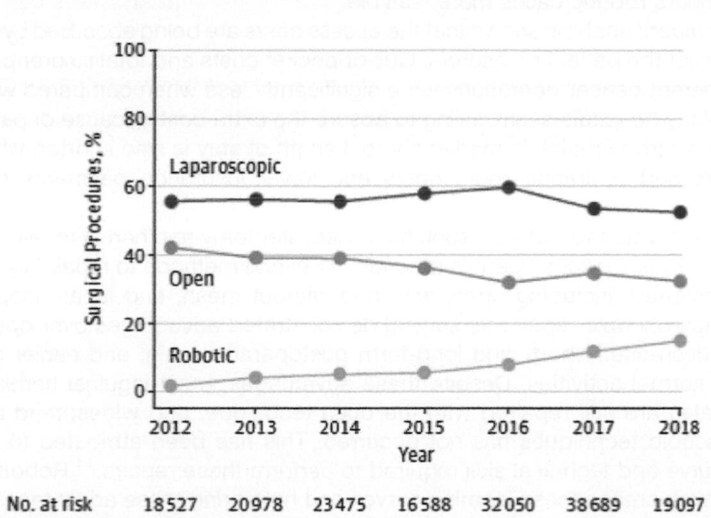

Fig. 1. The 2012 to 2018 temporal trends in the proportional use of robotic, laparoscopic, and open surgery. (*From* Sheetz KH, Claflin J, Dimick JB. Trends in the adoption of robotic surgery for common surgical procedures. JAMA Netw Open. 2020;3(1):e1918911; with permission.)

to the patient, if surgical conditions, such as refractory reflux or colon cancer, are identified but must be referred elsewhere for treatment.

Rural hospitals already have difficulty attracting talented, young surgeons because of the perception of an undesirable location, reduced reimbursement, lack of peer support, sense of isolation, and limited call coverage.[8] Teaching programs are more likely to be located in high-volume urban centers, which are more likely to use robotics technology.[7] Newer graduates who have trained on the technology may shy away from hospitals where it is not available.[10] In a recent survey of community general surgery residents, 77% believed robotics would be important in the future, and 63% believed that robotics would be important to their particular career.[11]

The increased cost of robotic surgery is the principle criticism of the technology. A rural hospital with limited financial resources may not be able to afford to adopt such an expensive technology. Cost of ownership of a robotics system includes several fixed and variable cost components. Fixed costs include the initial purchase of the machine ($1.5–2 million) plus yearly service contract ($154,000). Variable costs include disposable supplies, implants, operating room time, and personnel. Analysis of these data demonstrates varying costs per case from $4309 for cholecystectomy to $17,970 for rectal resection.[12]

The case volume effect on the fixed costs is highly significant. The more cases that are done the larger the decrease in the fixed cost per case. With increased volumes, surgeons and staff become more efficient with time and supplies, further decreasing costs per case.[12] This is an important consideration for rural hospitals where a modest number of annual cases (~300) may not be achievable by a single surgeon. Multiple surgeons and/or specialties will likely be required to make a robotics program financially viable in the rural setting. Not only higher volumes, but increased efficiency decreases costs. Surgeon efficiency increases with time and case volume. Maintaining efficient staff is equally important. Depending on the particular rural hospital a dedicated smaller group may make it easier to maintain efficiency, whereas high staff turnover can create efficiency problems. A smaller staff may even make urgent add-ons and after hours robotic cases more feasible.

Another recent analysis shows that the excess costs are being absorbed by the hospitals, and not the patient or insurers. Out-of-pocket costs and total insurer payments for five different cancer operations were significantly less when compared with open surgery. Many hospitals seem willing to absorb the extra cost because of patient demand and desire to maintain market share. Length of stay is also shorter, which may make increased operating room costs and lower insurance payments easier to absorb.[7]

Bread and butter procedures, such as cholecystectomy and hernia repair, make up a large portion of a rural surgeon's practice.[13] Several methods to repair inguinal hernia are accepted, including open, with and without mesh, and laparoscopic techniques. Laparoscopic repair has several demonstrated advantages over open repair including decreased short- and long-term postoperative pain, and earlier return to work and normal activities. Despite these advantages, most inguinal hernias in the United States are still repaired with the open technique, and widespread adoption of laparoscopic techniques has not occurred. This has been attributed to the long learning curve and technical skill required to perform these repairs.[14] Robotics technology may decrease these learning curves and help bring these advantages to rural communities.

Evidence is beginning to emerge regarding advantages in cholecystectomy. There is evidence to suggest that rate of conversion to open surgery and bile duct injuries are lower with robotic cholecystectomy, and intraoperative fluorescent cholangiography in the elective and acute setting.[15] Additionally, intraoperative fluorescent cholangiography is ideal for the rural setting because it is interpreted real time by the surgeon, requires no additional personal to perform, and radiologic interpretation is not necessary. Use of the robot on common surgeries, such as hernia and gallbladder, may also serve as a bridge to more complex surgeries.

Another important part of a rural general surgeon's practice is colorectal surgery. Some evidence is beginning to emerge in the colorectal literature. Robotic colorectal surgery is safe and feasible when compared with laparoscopy. Conversion to open procedures is lower with robotic surgery, and although not statistically significant there was a trend toward lower anastomotic leak rates, negative margins, and preservation of autonomic function. Especially important to the rural general surgeon, where case volumes may not be as high, is a decreased learning curve compared with laparoscopic surgery.[16] Again, this may allow the rural surgeon to keep and operate on patients locally rather than feeling the need to send them out for treatment.

Further research is needed to determine difference in costs and benefits of robotic-assisted surgery, especially in a rural environment. Complications, readmissions, reoperation, days in hospital, costs, and quality-of-life measures should all be taken into account when evaluating the effectiveness of robotic technology. Regionalization, recruitment, and economic factors will determine whether robotics technology is appropriate to adopt for a particular rural community. Although initial reports favored laparoscopic surgery because of financial concerns, more recent reports indicate that robotic technology is comparable and in some cases better than laparoscopic approaches. In addition, the inherent benefits of the advanced technology of robotic surgery are readily apparent to those who have used it, making robotic surgery the minimally invasive surgery of choice for many surgeons. As the costs of robotic technology decrease because of increased vendor competition in the robotic market, it is the opinion of the authors that robotic surgery will replace many current laparoscopic procedures in the next 10 to 15 years. These same declines in cost will make robotic surgery more available for rural hospitals and surgeons. Much research and development is occurring in the robotic surgery arena, which will continue to enhance robotic surgery platforms and allow all surgeons and patients to benefit from these advances. Rural surgeons should be able to take advantage of these advances, as do their urban and academic counterparts.

Magnetic Sphincter Augmentation

Another area of medicine that has seen a myriad of new technologies and interventions in the past three decades is the management of gastroesophageal reflux disease (GERD). In addition to medical treatment with proton pump inhibitors (PPI) and H_2 receptor antagonists, developed and marketed between the late 1970s and 2010, endoscopic and operative technologies and procedures have been developed to manage and prevent GERD and its sequelae. With the advent of laparoscopic minimally invasive antireflux procedures in the 1990s, operative therapy became a more attractive option. As the adverse effects of long-term medical management of GERD have become known, other methods to manage GERD have been developed. Magnetic sphincter augmentation (MSA) is a new addition to the armamentarium of the general surgeon for the treatment of this condition.

Gastroesophageal reflux is a common problem throughout the world with an estimated prevalence of between 10% and 30% in westernized countries.[17] Although the first choice of therapy for GERD is generally medical with PPI and lifestyle modifications, approximately 30% to 40% of patients report persistent symptoms despite optimized PPI therapy.[18] The gold standard of surgical treatment of refractory GERD is the Nissen fundoplication.[18] Randomized controlled trials have shown that the Nissen fundoplication provides superior resolution of reflux in the appropriate patient population.[19]

MSA technology involves a series of magnetic beads interconnected with a titanium wire. It is placed laparoscopically around the gastroesophageal junction and applies a magnetic force to keep the lower esophageal sphincter closed. The device allows for passage of a bolus of food during swallowing and subsequently releases during elevated intragastric pressure and allows for belching or vomiting.[17] It is indicated in nonobese patients with GERD confirmed on 24-hour pH monitoring and symptoms despite maximized medical therapy. This is typically performed on patients who have a hiatal hernia smaller than 3 cm. Rona and colleagues[20] and Buckley and colleagues[21] reviewed the MSA efficacy on patients with larger hiatal hernias (≥5 cm) and found similar outcomes to those with smaller hiatal hernia.

A meta-analysis in *Surgical Endoscopy* identified three studies. They compared MSA with laparoscopic Nissen fundoplication (LNF). The significant findings showed MSA was superior in a patient's ability to belch and vomit. There were no differences between MSA and LNF in postoperative dysphagia, PPI elimination, and gas/bloating. There were more postoperative dilations required in the MSA group versus the LNF group. Overall morbidity profile was similar in both groups.[17,19]

MSA tends to have a shorter operative time and is technically easier to perform than LNF.[17,19] Postoperative complications with MSA placement include: significant dysphagia requiring removal (0.5%–8.3%), device failure or erosion into the esophagus (0.1%–1.2%), and readmission to hospital within 30 days (1.3%–5.4%).[22] MSA is proving to be efficacious in the treatment of medically refractory GERD, but more data need to be collected to determine the long-term efficacy of MSA when in comparison with the gold standard LNF.

MSA can be performed in rural settings and offers the surgeon and patient an additional option to treat refractory GERD. If the surgeon is appropriately trained and feels comfortable placing an MSA device, they should add this operation to their armamentarium. There are no data showing that an MSA placed in rural settings has outcomes that are different than those placed in urban centers. This procedure is an example of a new technology that is available and appropriate for the rural surgeon. This can benefit the rural community and hospital by providing new and advanced technology in a rural setting.

Gastrointestinal Endoscopy

Gastrointestinal endoscopy is a key component of most rural surgeons' practice, comprising between 40% and 60% of their practices.[13,23] As in minimally invasive surgery, technologic advances have improved endoscopic methods and capabilities in recent years. A summary of many of the new technologies in gastrointestinal endoscopy is shown in **Table 1**. Many of the listed advanced technologies in **Table 1** require advanced training, significant financial investment, and a steady volume of patients with a specific diagnosis. These conditions are generally not present in a rural hospital making it impractical for their use by a rural surgeon. Several of these technologies are more appropriate for tertiary referral centers (eg, chromoendoscopy, endomicroscopy, endoscopic ultrasound, endoscopic transoral therapies, endoscopic mucosal resection, transient elastography, single- and double-balloon enteroscopy), but some may be advantageous and useful for rural surgeons (eg, endoscopic closure devices, endosuturing devices, radiofrequency ablation). Nonetheless, rural surgeons should be familiar with these technologic advances because in select cases they may be of significant benefit for the patient and warrant referral. Additionally, it is also beneficial for a rural surgeon to be knowledgeable of these technologies because rural patients

Table 1
Advanced technology in endoscopy

Technology	Description	Advantage
Advanced endoscopic imaging	High-definition and magnification endoscopes (endomicroscopy) with electronic chromoendoscopy	Improved accuracy in diagnosis and biopsy of mucosal lesions and polyps at microscopic level
Endoscopic ultrasound	Sonographic identification and characterization of cystic and solid lesions, ultrasound-directed biopsy, and internal drainage of fluid collections	More accurate diagnosis of solid and cystic lesions before surgery, avoidance of surgery for some lesions, improved staging of malignancies
Radiofrequency ablation	Eradication of superficial mucosal lesions using radiofrequency energy	Noninvasive eradication of Barrett's esophagus, prevention of progression to malignancy
Endoscopic transoral therapies	Peroral endoscopic lower esophageal sphincter myotomy for achalasia, peroral endoscopic pyloric myotomy for gastroparesis, peroral endoscopic septum division for Zenker diverticulum	Correction and management of disorders of submucosal layers of gastrointestinal tract without need for invasive open or laparoscopic surgical procedures
Natural orifice transluminal endoscopic surgery	Endoscopic intra-abdominal surgery through natural orifice (transoral, transvaginal, transanal) to remove diseased organ (appendix, gallbladder, kidney, mesorectum)	Intra-abdominal surgery without surgical incision, postoperative pain, or scarring
Endoscopic mucosal resection, endoscopic submucosal dissection techniques	Techniques and instrumentation to lift mucosa and dissect in submucosal plane to separate and remove lesions that do not penetrate submucosa	Resect large polyps or early malignancies without invasive surgical procedure
Endoscopic closure devices, endosuturing devices	Endoscopic devices to close created openings, fistulas, or perforations of the gastrointestinal tract	Repair and closure of opening of gastrointestinal tract without open or laparoscopic surgery
Transient elastography	Noninvasive means to evaluate degree of liver fibrosis	Avoid complications of percutaneous biopsy of liver
Single- and double-balloon enteroscopy	Small bowel mucosa visualization and assessment	Improved accuracy of current small bowel assessment methods

may have them performed at a tertiary center and return to their rural community for further care. Knowledge of the technology and its purpose may allow the rural surgeon to diagnose and manage some post-procedure symptoms or complications. Although some may argue that these technologies are encroaching on the current standards of treatment of basic general surgical diseases (eg, natural orifice transluminal endoscopic surgery, peroral endoscopic myotomy), the current results, technologic requirements, steep learning curves, and validation of benefits of these technologies has not resulted in widespread acceptance and use. As the technologies improve and the ability to perform more complex procedures through an endoscope evolve, rural surgeons who are already facile with endoscopic techniques may find that incorporation of select advanced endoscopic technologies has the potential to benefit their practices and communities. The adoption of any of these new technologies by a rural surgeon requires collaboration between the rural surgeon (training and certification) and his or her rural facility (acquisition of the necessary equipment and staff training) to enable the technology to be used at that facility.

TELEMEDICINE

Another area of technology that has changed and will continue to change the practice of medicine is telemedicine or telehealth. The definition of telemedicine varies according to the source and includes: the use of electronic information and telecommunications technologies to support and promote long-distance clinical health care, patient and professional health-related education, and public health and health administration (Health Resources and Services Administration of the US Department of Health and Human Services); the practice of medicine when the doctor and patient are widely separated using two-way voice and visual communication (Merriam-Webster Dictionary); and any form of medical practice in which diagnostic information is transmitted for analysis by a physician, who performs teleconsultation (medical-dictionary.thefreedictionary.com).

Telemedicine technology is particularly useful in rural communities because its primary purpose is to connect health care providers, patients, and other health care professionals over long distances. The technology has a wide variety of uses and currently is being used for many health care applications ranging from long distance pathologic analysis to monitoring and management of intensive care unit patients (**Table 2**). Although the detailed discussion of telemedicine technology and the wide variety of applications within this field is beyond the scope of this article, the current principle uses are listed in the **Table 2**. One of the most obvious advantages of many of the current telemedicine applications is the ability to bring a specific specialty service to a location where it is not available. The unavailability of specialty and subspecialty services is common in rural communities and is caused by several factors including remote location, low population, intermittent need, difficulty in recruitment, inability to support the specialty, or financial shortcomings of the location. Because these factors are present in many rural locations, telemedicine applications are ideal for rural hospitals. The ability to bring specialty physicians and patients together over long distances is beneficial in many ways including saving travel time, travel expenses, increasing convenience, and significantly improved cost-effectiveness for the rural facility. In addition to direct clinical interactions between members of the health care team, telehealth technology is used for education, consultation, monitoring, administrative meetings, and research.

Almost all telemedicine technology requires the use of the Internet and many require high-speed Internet to accommodate the large amounts of data that are transmitted.

Table 2
Telemedicine applications

Application	Specialty	Use
Teleradiology	Radiology	Interpretation of diagnostic imaging studies by qualified radiologists from long distances
eICU	Intensive care	Continuous remote monitoring of critical care patients by intensivists, multiple facilities can be monitored by one eICU support center
Telehealth	General medicine	Primary care evaluations for new and follow-up patients, management of some basic medical problems without direct face-to-face encounters
Telepathology	Pathology	Transfer of pathology image data between distant locations for the purposes of diagnosis, education, and research
Telecardiology	Cardiology	Remote diagnosis and treatment of heart disease, including ECG, Holter monitors, pacemaker monitoring, arrhythmias, coronary artery disease, CHF, sudden cardiac arrest
Telemedicine follow-up	Multiple	Use of telecommunications technology for follow-up after hospital or clinic visits for patients from remote distances
Telenursing	Nursing	Home health, home nursing care, and advice
Teleconferencing	Multiple	Conferencing between multiple facilities or providers for review of patient cases (eg, tumor boards), clinical, educational, and administrative meetings
Teledermatology	Dermatology	Diagnoses, consultation, and treatment of skin conditions and tumors of the skin over a distance using audio, visual, and data communication
Telepharmacy	Pharmacy	Delivery of pharmaceutical care to patients in locations where direct contact with a pharmacist is not available
Telepsychiatry	Psychiatry	The delivery of psychiatric assessments, care, and counseling through telecommunications technology (videoconferencing)

Abbreviations: CHF, congestive heart failure; ECG, electrocardiogram; eICU, electronic intensive care unit.

As more and more rural facilities and homes gain access to high-speed Internet many more telemedicine applications will be available in rural communities. Additionally, the widespread use of smartphones with their data transmission capability and enhanced video features has facilitated several telemedicine applications for patients at home. Currently almost all hospitals, including rural critical access hospitals, use some form of telemedicine technology, and in many cases are dependent on it for their continued existence and function.

As with other technologies, in addition to the benefits of telemedicine technologies, there are also barriers and problems with the implementation and use of these technologies. Barriers to telemedicine technology include the cost of the hardware and software; regulatory requirements from local, state, and national bodies; billing and coding uncertainties; licensing requirements for the health care providers and institution; and the need to safeguard patient confidentiality and meet HIPAA requirements. Additionally, the medicolegal implications of long distance health care are not always evident and may not be covered by the liability insurance of the physician and hospital. Despite these barriers the significant advantages of telemedicine capabilities have made this an important and essential part of most health care institutions, especially in rural hospitals.

Many telemedicine applications are designed for primary care and nonprocedural specialists but there are uses that can be adapted for surgeons. For instance, in postoperative situations for patients who live a significant distance from the hospital, the ability to communicate and even visualize wounds through smartphone cameras can save the surgeon and the patient time, unnecessary travel, and expense. Additionally, the use of telemedicine for consultations between the rural surgeon and their primary referring partner is helpful in several situations including trauma, intraoperative decisions, complex case management, and decisions on the timing and availability of transfer.

DISCUSSION

Advanced technology has changed medicine and surgery drastically over the past few decades in rural and urban locations. In rural hospitals select advanced technologies can alleviate some of the difficulties in rural practices while providing benefits to the surgeon, hospital, and rural community. Some advanced technologies may not be appropriate for rural hospitals for several reasons, but cost, necessary training, and adequate patient volumes are principle concerns. Most new technologies are tested in academic centers and the choice of when and if they are appropriate for rural hospitals can be made after the validation and consequences of the technology are better known. In general, most patients in rural and urban areas would prefer to get their health care closer to home. Patients in rural communities are more knowledgeable, in many cases because of their ability to research their health care conditions on the Internet. Rather than seek out advanced technologies in distant locations, most would be happy to have access to some forms of advanced technology in their own rural hospitals.

The introduction of new technologies into surgical practice has been historically met with skepticism, steep learning curves, and varied levels of adoption.[24] The current deluge of new technologies in surgery and medicine are no exception. The rural surgeon has a unique opportunity to review and evaluate new surgical technologies that are developed in urban medical centers and become the primary driving force in bringing them to his or her rural hospital if they are deemed to be worthwhile, cost-effective, and beneficial. Many of the motivations for hospitals in more competitive environments to quickly acquire and endorse new technologies may not be present in rural hospitals. This can allow the rural surgeon to wait until the technology is fully evaluated for safety, cost-effectiveness, and outcomes before deciding on bringing the technology to their practice. Judicious and intelligent decision making regarding the adoption of new technologies in rural locations can reap significant benefit to the surgeon, hospital, and community. The adoption of new technologies in rural communities must be individualized based on the capabilities, resources, and needs of the rural surgeon and hospital.

It is inevitable that there will continue to be new technologies developed and marketed in surgery and medicine. Many emerging technologies are currently in development, such as artificial intelligence, genetically based treatment programs, health information exchanges, miniaturized surgical interventions, and others. The possibilities are limitless and mind boggling. Rural surgeons can and should be at the forefront of the decisions for the adoption and use of advanced technologies in their communities.

DISCLOSURE

The authors have nothing to disclose.

REFERENCES

1. Stefanidis D, Fanelli RD, Price R, et al. Guidelines for the introduction of new technology and techniques. Available at: https://www.sages.org/publications/guidelines/guidelines-introduction-new-technology-techniques/. Accessed March 15, 2020.
2. McCulloch P, Altman DG, Campbell WB, et al. No surgical innovation without evaluation: the IDEAL recommendations. Lancet 2009;374:1105–12.
3. Biffl WL, Spain DA, Reitsma AM, et al. Responsible development and application of surgical innovations: a position statement of the Society of University Surgeons. J Am Coll Surg 2008;206:1204–9.
4. American College of Surgeons. Statements on emerging surgical technologies and the evaluation of credentials. Bull Am Coll Surg 1994;79:40–1.
5. Herron DM, Marohn M, SAGES-MIRA Robotic Surgery Consensus Group. A consensus document on robotic surgery. Surg Endosc 2008;22(2):313–25.
6. Sheetz KH, Claflin J, Dimick JB. Trends in the adoption of robotic surgery for common surgical procedures. JAMA Netw Open 2020;3(1):e1918911.
7. Nabi J, Friedlander DF, Chen X, et al. Assessment of out-of-pocket costs for robotic cancer surgery in US adults. JAMA Netw Open 2020;3(1):e1919185.
8. Antonenko DR. Rural surgery: the North Dakota experience. Surg Clin North Am 2009;89(6):1367.
9. McCollister HM, Severson PA, LeMieur TP, et al. Building and maintaining a successful surgery program in rural Minnesota. Surg Clin North Am 2009;89(6):1349, ix.
10. Zender J, Thell C. Developing a successful robotic surgery program in a rural hospital. AORN J 2010;92(1):72–86.
11. Krause W, Bird J. The importance of robotic-assisted procedures in residency training to applicants of a community general surgery residency program. J Robot Surg 2019;13(3):379–82 [Erratum appears in J Robot Surg. 2018 Oct 16].
12. Feldstein J, Schwander B, Roberts M, et al. Cost of ownership assessment for a da Vinci robot based on US real-world data. Int J Med Robot 2019;15:e2023.

13. Harris JD, Hosford CC, Sticca RP. A comprehensive analysis of surgical procedures in rural surgery practices. Am J Surg 2010;200(6):820–6.
14. Iraniha A, Peloquin J. Long-term quality of life and outcomes following robotic assisted TAPP inguinal hernia repair. J Robot Surg 2018;12(2):261–9.
15. Gangemi A, Danilkowicz R, Elli FE, et al. Could ICG-aided robotic cholecystectomy reduce the rate of open conversion reported with laparoscopic approach? A head to head comparison of the largest single institution studies. J Robot Surg 2017;11(1):77–82.
16. Aly EH. Robotic colorectal surgery: summary of the current evidence. Int J Colorectal Dis 2014;29(1):1–8.
17. Schizas D, Mastoraki A, Papoutsi E, et al. LINX® reflux management system to bridge the "treatment gap" in gastroesophageal reflux disease: a systematic review of 35 studies. World J Clin Cases 2020;8(2):294–305.
18. Skubleny D, Switzer NJ, Dang J, et al. LINX® magnetic esophageal sphincter augmentation versus Nissen fundoplication for gastroesophageal reflux disease: a systematic review and meta-analysis. Surg Endosc 2017;31:3078–84.
19. Lundell L, Miettinen P, Myrvold HE, et al. Comparison of outcomes twelve years after antireflux surgery or omeprazole maintenance therapy for reflux esophagitis. Clin Gastroenterol Hepatol 2009;7:1292–8.
20. Rona KA, Reynolds J, Schwameis K, et al. Efficacy of magnetic sphincter augmentation in patients with large hiatal hernias. Surg Endosc 2017;31: 2096–102.
21. Buckley FP, Bell RCW, Freeman K, et al. Favorable results from a prospective-evaluation of 200 patients with large hiatal hernias undergoing LINX magnetic sphincter augmentation. Surg Endosc 2018;32:1762–8.
22. Kirkham EN, Main BG, Jones KJ, et al. Systemic review of the introduction and evaluation of magnetic augmentation of the lower oesophageal sphincter for gastro-oesphageal reflux disease. Br J Surg 2020;107:44–55.
23. Sticca RP, Mullin BC, Harris JD, et al. Surgical specialty procedures in rural surgery practices: implications for rural surgery training. Am J Surg 2012;204(6): 1007–12.
24. Wilson CB. Adoption of new surgical technology. BMJ 2006;332(7533):112–4.

Dealing with the Sick Rural Surgery Patient in Need of Transfer

Julie Conyers, MD, MBA

KEYWORDS

• Rural surgery • Interhospital transfer • Outcomes • Patient handoffs

KEY POINTS

- The interhospital transfer process is largely understudied in the United States and practices vary widely.
- Interhospital transfer status is associated with worse outcomes.
- The handoff process during interhospital and intrahospital transport often is incomplete.
- Evidence supports stabilization or even damage or source control for hemorrhage or sepsis prior to transfer.

INTRODUCTION

By virtue of their location, rural surgeons practice in low-resource environments, often without direct access to specialists or other ancillary services. The resources and scope of practice vary with each rural location and often are dynamic. In other words, resources may change from day to day or from week to week. For instance, a facility may need to transfer a ventilated patient, because only 1 respiratory therapist is available, or a hemodynamically unstable patient may require transfer to obtain an echocardiogram. From a resource standpoint, rural medicine may demonstrate more breadth but no depth beyond the singular. Although rural surgeons have chosen to practice in wide open spaces, they understand the feeling of isolation when standing next to their sick patient in need of transfer. Rural surgeons may on occasion need to transfer an emergent case, because they have been overburdened by weeks of consecutive call or because a solo rural surgeon may not be in town for the postoperative care.

The care for the urban or rural surgical patient is increasingly more complex, since the establishment of intensive care unit (ICUs) in the 1950s. The 2009 Nationwide Inpatient Sample identified 1,397,712 transferred patients and 39,692,211 nontransfer

Department of Surgery, PeaceHealth Ketchikan, 3100 Tongass Avenue, Ketchikan, AK 99901, USA
E-mail address: jconyers@peacehealth.org

Surg Clin N Am 100 (2020) 921–936
https://doi.org/10.1016/j.suc.2020.06.009 **surgical.theclinics.com**
0039-6109/20/

patients when comparing the characteristics and outcomes of each category.[1] Not only did this study find that transfer patients have inferior outcomes compared with nontransfer patients, but also it described that approximately 1.4 million patients experienced interhospital transfers (IHTs) in 2009. Approximately 4.8% of index encounters result in IHTs, with the highest rates for patients living in rural areas, ranging from 9.8% to 10.1%.[2] Too often rural surgeons find themselves at the bedside of a sick patient in need of transfer for escalation of care without a fluid or even standardized process to facilitate the transfer. Furthermore, the Critical Access Hospital (CAH) 96-hour rule requires physicians to certify that Medicare beneficiaries may reasonably be expected to be discharged or transferred to another hospital within 96 hours. Transfer of these patients delays their care and adds to the total cost for patients who are appropriate for that facility. Given the author's location in an archipelago of more than 1100 islands in southeast Alaska, such transfers incur a bill ranging from $70,000 to $90,000 secondary to the requirement of fixed-wing transports of distances no less than 670 miles. **Fig. 1** illustrates the location of Ketchikan, Alaska, relative to the United States and Canada. Regulatory and organizational pressures often result in the transfer decisions and destinations contrary to a patient's goals.

THE PARADOX

Consistent with other wealthy countries, the United States has developed a specialized health care system. The mismatch between patient needs and hospital resources, however, is not uncommon. Specialized services are distributed unevenly. Approximately 1 in 20 Medicare patients experience an ICU to ICU transfer. Nguyen and colleagues[3] have proposed 3 possibilities to address the mismatch parody:

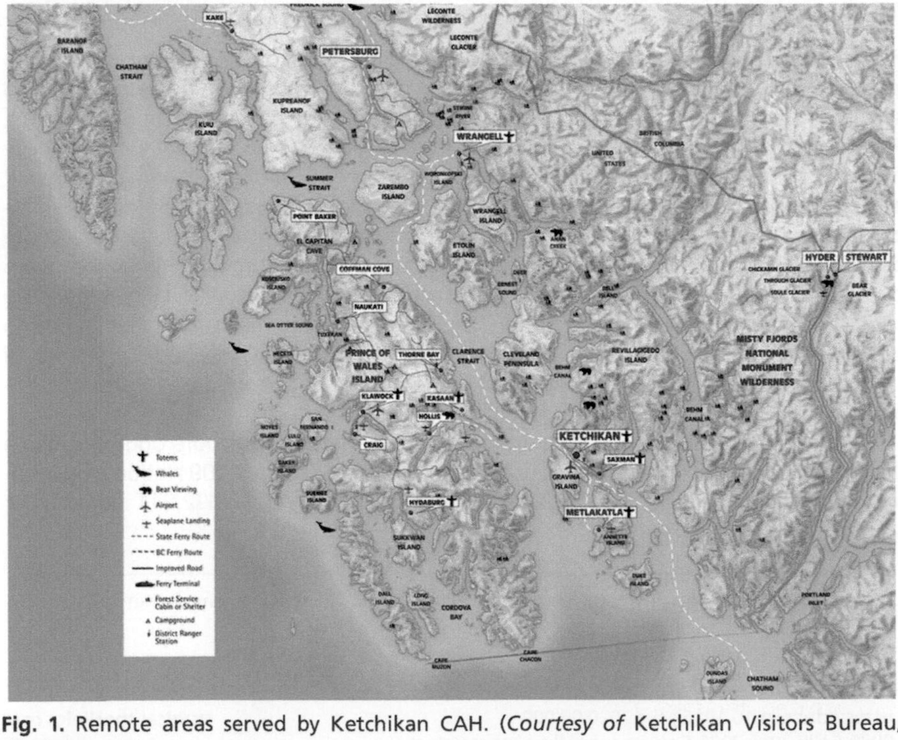

Fig. 1. Remote areas served by Ketchikan CAH. (*Courtesy of* Ketchikan Visitors Bureau, Ketchikan, AK.)

- Move the patient to the expertise
- Move the expertise to the patient
- Expertise everywhere

Tiered Regionalization: Move the Patient to the Expertise

The American College of Surgeons (ACS) models of trauma and cancer care already have shown the benefits of tiered regionalized systems. Identifying ICU referral centers within regions according to location, resources, and performance with oversight by professional societies is similar to ACS models. Tiered regionalization exists in trauma systems and has shown benefit.

Telemedicine: Move the Expertise to the Patient

In today's world, technology rarely is a barrier to telemedicine. It does require a capital investment that is not negligible in the context of critical care. In rural medicine, it can help to bridge the resource mismatch and distance gap, but the utilization is surprisingly low. Outcome studies have ranged from improved to no effect. It cannot substitute for intubation or central lines, but those procedures are not a barrier to the rural surgeon. Liability and licensure are concerns, but perhaps the biggest barrier is poor reimbursement. For calendar year 2018, the Medicare payment amount for Healthcare Common Procedure Coding System code Q3014 (telehealth originating site facility fee) is 80% of the lesser of the actual charge, or $25.76.[4] In the author's practice environment, keeping the patient close to home and saving the 670-mile transfer cost demonstrates a significant return on investment for the US health care system. The maximum facility charge of $25.76 does not cover costs to implement telemedicine at the originating site when taking into consideration the personnel costs to support this model.

Regional Outreach: Expertise Everywhere

The expertise everywhere strategy involves cooperation by all hospitals regardless of size to increase the quality of care. Nguyen and colleagues[3] describe a relatively small investment in infrastructure. The concept proposes facilitating benchmarking across all sites while providing data to individual hospitals relative to the benchmarks. Shared resources would be used to target quality improvement. This model assumes all stakeholders have aligned incentives and answer to the same master. Competing health care systems are unlikely to embrace this sort of cooperation. Rigorous data gathering and benchmarking in low-volume, rural hospitals are met with resource challenges and interpretation of small data sets.

THE TRANSFER PROCESS

Bosk and colleagues[5] have studied the IHT process both qualitatively and quantitatively. They identified 4 components of the transfer process:

1. Identifying transfer-eligible patients
2. Identifying a destination
3. Negotiating the transfer
4. Accomplishing the transfer

Triage

Protocolized transfers for conditions, such as ST-segment elevation myocardial infarction resulted in a more fluid process. Conditions without protocols, however, often are described as cumbersome and often fraught with ambiguity and disagreements in the transfer process. Emergency department (ED) physicians may find themselves caught between the local service refusal to admit, and the receiving hospital asserting patients should not be transferred. Clinicians who practice in a low-resource environment also consider the impact of Emergency Medical Treatment and Labor Act (EMTALA) on their ability to transfer in the triage process. EMTALA overwhelmingly focuses on emergency care rather than IHT of critically ill patients. Furthermore, EMTALA also includes a nondiscrimination provision, also known as "the reverse dumping provision." This provision imposes a duty on receiving hospitals to accept appropriate transfers based on 2 caveats: (1) the receiving hospital must have specialized capabilities or facilities and (2) must have the capacity to treat the patient.[6] An example may be the ground fall of an elderly patient on aspirin with findings of intracranial blood on CT and who is felt to be a low risk for rebleeding by neurosurgery. Admitting this patient without a care plan or nursing expertise may result in a poor outcome. Moreover, if a patient deteriorates, EMTALA no longer applies, and clinicians find themselves begging and/or shopping for an accepting physician at a receiving facility. At the author's facility in SE Alaska, the minimum decision-to-arrival time is 4.5 hours, with an average time between 6 hours to 8 hours, provided there is a plane on the ground. Reverse-dumping provisions do not apply to the inpatient scenario. For instance, after 3 weeks of refusals, the author's facility finally found an acceptance for an admitted traumatic brain injury patient.

Transfers often are insurance-mandated, but the liability of transfer is a burden of the physicians. The physician must document that the benefits of IHT outweigh the risks often without a complete understanding of a patient's condition due to limited resources. Also, there seems to be a gray area in liability once the handoff has occurred to the transfer team. On occasion, a physician at a small hospital may not have resources to stabilize a patient and must transfer to definitive care for any hope of survival. The decision to transfer often is determined by the rural hospital's capability to treat possible complications and proximity to a referral center, as discussed in the previous example.

Destination

Bosk and colleagues described conditions with protocols for transfer often were determined by institutional arrangements. Destination may be dictated by formal ownership or cultivated relationships between physicians. What would surprise the general public is that quality indicators in this qualitative study did not influence destination decisions. The investigators also noted that patient-centered factors were of little influence in the destination choice. Insurance also played a role in destination, often slowing the process and even routing the patient to a more distant hospital but not necessarily a superior hospital.

Negotiating the Transfer

When standing at the bedside of an unstable patient, many rural surgeons are too familiar with the string of phone calls to convince an acceptance or simply find a bed. Often the implication is that the rural hospital is incompetent or lazy. The bureaucratic process can be a nightmare on the sending end keeping physicians by phone rather than at the bedside of the sick patient. A refusal after a 30-minute wait for a return call results in starting over again. Understandably, flight crews do not deploy without an accepting facility. Identifying an accepting facility is a relief, but interacting with a supportive, helpful accepting physician underscores the importance of fostering relationships with referral centers.

Accomplishing the Transfer

Distance, terrain, water, weather, local resources, timeliness, and condition of the patient all influence this process making each rural facility unique. Should the patient go by ground or air? Does the community have paramedics or voluntary emergency medical services (EMS)? Does the patient need a critical care transport crew? Is the weather too hostile to travel by air or can EMS go by ground? When is the transport team be expected to arrive? What is the expected door-to-door time? Does the transport team have or need blood? In rural facilities, prehospital transport often is aided by Good Samaritans, civilian search and rescue teams, or search and rescue by the National Guard or the Coast Guard, often taking many hours in harsh conditions. In very remote rural areas, there is no golden hour but rather a golden day.

In Ketchikan, Alaska, a ferry (day or night) must take the patient by ambulance across the channel to the island where the airport is located. All transfers are by fixed-wing aircraft. Some patients must travel by water, ground, and air to reach the CAH, with paramedic-staffed EMS available only for the last leg of transport. For example, a floatplane transporting tourists crashed into a mountain on a remote island in July of 2018. All 11 survivors were rescued by a Coast Guard helicopter (basket hoist) off the mountain and then transported to a logging camp. The survivors then were transported by industrial helicopters to the island.

OUTCOMES OF INTERHOSPITAL TRANSFER PATIENTS

Transfers of a rural, critically ill patient is based on the assumption that the transfer likely will result in a decrease in morbidity and mortality as opposed to staying in the rural facility. Should rural surgeons challenge the conventional wisdom that rural ICU to urban ICU transfers unquestionably add benefit? For conditions, such as acute coronary syndrome, stroke, and trauma, previous studies have shown protocolized IHT benefits outweigh the risks. Surprisingly, little empirical evidence supports this assumption for other conditions. A retrospective data analysis by Rush and colleagues[7] of the Nationwide Readmissions Database from 22 states examined mortality and length of stay of IHT for a total of 1630 septic, mechanically ventilated patients compared with a propensity-matched non-IHT cohort of 1630 patients. After propensity matching, IHT was not associated with a difference in mortality, but IHT was associated with longer length of stay.[7] This study acknowledged the limitations of administrative data and the lack of many variables in the care of these sick patients. Also, details of the originating hospital, the receiving hospital, and transfers themselves were not available. This study does raise the question, however, of whether the transfer process harms some patients (discussed later).

Interhospital Transfer Status Associated with Increased Mortality

Although prospective, randomized data regarding outcomes of IHT on the rural surgery patient are rare or nonexistent, 1 variable associated with increased mortality in the surgical ICU was IHT status, as reported by Arthur and colleagues.[8] These patients were found to be older and sicker. Mortality rates for IHT patients were highest on the emergency surgery (18%), transplant surgery (16%), and gastrointestinal surgery (8%) services.[8]

Interhospital Transfer Associated with Delay of Definitive Surgery

Numerous retrospective studies confirm the delay in definitive surgical intervention of IHT patients as expected. Limmer and colleagues[9] from Sydney, Australia, looked at time to surgical intervention of IHT patients from a local nearby district hospital (Hospital B) with a mean transit of only 28 minutes by ground compared with directly admitted patients to a large metropolitan hospital in New South Wales (Hospital A) over 1 year. Hospital B performs predominantly elective surgery, so a vast majority of emergency cases are transferred to Hospital A. Of the 910 patients who underwent emergency surgery for abdominal pain in 2013, 290 patients were transferred from Hospital B to Hospital A. Time to surgical intervention was a mean 46.9 hours for IHT patients compared with a mean 32.7 hours for directly admitted patients ($P<.001$) to Hospital A. Transferred patients spent a mean 8.1 hours in the receiving hospital ED. Time to surgery for perforated peptic ulcer was not statistically different for transferred versus direct admit patients. Overall length of stay was 6.2 days for transfer patients and 4.6 days for direct admit patients ($P<.001$). This study demonstrates the significant delay in emergency surgery despite short transport times in an integrated health care system. Increasing transport times by hours in a fragmented health care system only lengthens the delay of emergent surgical intervention.

Desai and colleagues[10] reviewed all patients with hip fractures admitted to a Level I trauma center in Canada between 2005 and 2012. A total of 890 patients met inclusion criteria with 715 directly admitted patients and 175 patients who were transferred. Transferred patients' median delay from initial admission to operation was 93 hours. Directly admitted patients waited a median of 44 hours. Delays often were due the lack of beds at the receiving hospital. Median delay in transfer prior to policy changes was 47 hours and 27 hours after policy changes in this integrated health care system. Median length of stay was 20 days for transfer patients as opposed to 13 days for direct admit patients.[10]

Decline of Community General Surgeons?

A small study out of Portland, Maine, by Misercola and colleagues[11] published a retrospective chart review of 161 patients transferred to an acute care surgery service at a tertiary facility compared with 611 directly admitted patient who resided locally. Demographics, clinical presentation, and outcomes were assessed. Transferred patients were older, had more comorbidities, and required more resources than local patients. ICU admissions were 24% versus 6%, length of stay was 8.2 days versus 3.4 days, Medicare beneficiaries were 55% versus 34%, and privately insured were 26% versus 45%, respectively, for transferred versus local admissions. Unexpectedly, the investigators found that approximately half of transfer patients underwent basic surgical procedures or did not require an intervention. This finding raised the concern for the lack of general surgery resources in surrounding communities.

BE CAREFUL WHAT YOU WISH FOR?

A stunning *U.S. News* article, published on May 19, 2015, titled, *Hospitals Move to Limit Low-Volume Surgeries*, by Steve Sternberg, described that Dartmouth-Hitchcock Medical Center, Johns Hopkins Medicine, and the University of Michigan were planning to impose minimum volume standards by barring hospitals within their systems from performing certain procedures. Dr Birkmeyer of Dartmouth-Hitchcock Medical Center was quoted: "Low volume hobbyists are bad for patients and we have to stop them" and "You might think it's only a problems with very small hospitals that are trying to run with the big dogs."[12] Perhaps the intent of this forced constraint is that IHT to high-volume centers result in better outcomes.

Interhospital Transfers May Have an Impact on Quality Metrics at Academic Centers

As the volume debate regarding surgery and quality outcomes continues to rage, academic centers are now finding that IHTs are impacting their quality metrics and possible financial performance. Ironically, Johns Hopkins participated in a study looking at 2011 ACS National Surgical Quality Improvement Program database in evaluating surgical outcomes of 6197 IHT patients compared with 47,267 direct admissions.[13] IHT patients had more complex and a broader range of procedures. On adjusted analysis, IHT patients had a much higher risk of complications and mortality, longer length of stay, and higher risk of readmission. The article raised the concern of unfairly financially penalizing hospitals that frequently accept transfers due to perceived poorer outcomes.

Interhospital Transfer Patients Consume More Resources

Crippen and colleagues[14] from the Department of Surgery, University of Florida at Gainsville, presented similar findings of IHT patients when looking at mortality, length of stay, and cost from January 2010 to December 2012. From a database of more than 1.4 million patients, IHT patients were found to have higher mortality rates, longer mean length of stay, and higher mean total costs. Hence, IHT patients had poorer outcomes and consume more resources. These investigators recommended that academic medical centers and community hospitals develop collaborative programs to permit collective assessment and decisions for complicated surgical patients.

One obvious dilemma with IHTs is that definitive emergency surgery often is significantly delayed and may be 1 of the many factors adversely affecting outcomes—even for the "big dogs." In this context, it seems inconceivable to bar smaller hospitals from performing emergency lifesaving surgeries, or worse, expecting community surgeons to perform emergency surgeries that otherwise would be forbidden electively.

THE ROLE OF DAMAGE CONTROL IN RURAL SURGERY

Should rural surgeons consider damage control in severely injured patients in hemorrhagic shock or for source control in patients with abdominal or other sepsis prior to transfer? Damage control surgery dates back to at least World War II. The US Army surgical teams clearing the beaches of Normandy were instructed to perform only lifesaving surgery and defer others until they reached England. The US Army forward surgical teams are designed to operate on only the most severely injured patients, using only rapid resource–sparing surgical interventions. The military concept of damage control surgery has been adapted in civilian medicine.[15] The initial operation should be brief with temporary measures to control hemorrhaging and intestinal perforations or leakage of urine. Measures may include packing of hepatic injuries, ligation of injured bowel, shunts into transected arteries, and vacuum-assisted closure or other coverage of the abdomen. In remote locations with long transport times, source control of sepsis may improve survival using similar concepts. This concept has been extrapolated from military outcomes. The goal is to avoid the lethal self-propagating triad of hypothermia, coagulopathy, and acidosis.

Harwell and colleagues[16] recently looked at outcomes of rural trauma patients who underwent damage control laparotomy as a means of pretransfer stabilization. Retrospective review of 47 patients who were grouped into 3 categories: damage control laparotomy at a rural hospital, patients unstable during transport, and patients stable during transport with a subsequent laparotomy. Mortality was 14.3% for damage control laparotomy at a rural hospital, 75% for unstable transfer patients, and 3.3% for stable transfer patients ($P<.001$).[16] Although this was a small retrospective study, mortality was high for unstable patients at transfer. Damage control surgery in the rural setting may deserve further research and discussion.

A randomized, controlled single-center trial addressing damage control laparotomy is under way at a Level I trauma center in Texas. The study plans to enroll a total of 56 patients with 28 in each arm.[17] Because the context of this study is in the urban trauma setting, it may not help surgeons in rural, remote locations with limited blood products.

TRANSPORTING THE CRITICALLY ILL PATIENT

The demand for critical care and ICU beds has increased significantly over the past decades. The complex IHT process varies widely without standardization. Rural hospitals often are unable to meet the needs of sick, aging patients in limited ICUs. As a result, the rural surgeon is increasingly transferring critically ill patients in need of multiple organ support. The transfer of critically ill patients is likely to continue to escalate due to increasing regionalization and the aging population. The author's CAH often is at maximum capacity in the summer months, when more than 1.3 million tourists visit the island, many of whom are elderly with multiple comorbidities. Because ICU beds are in such demand at tertiary centers, rural hospitals often are waiting for an ICU bed to become available. Larger ICUs often find an outflow bottle neck because they are forced to keep noncritical patients in an ICU bed until a step-down bed becomes available. The rural critically ill patient is in line behind the immediate needs of the tertiary facility.

Studies since the 1970s have addressed safety concerns of transferring critically ill patients. Waddell and colleagues[18] concluded that earlier transfer, resuscitation before the transfer, continuing medical care during the transfer, and a slower, smoother journey benefited the sick patients. These principles still hold true. This study, however, only addressed ground transport. Air transport by rotary or fixed wing aircraft over long distances poses challenges as well. Transport guidelines emerged in the 1990s to improve safety. A review by Waydhas,[19] published in 1999, reported that adverse events still occurred in up to 70% of transports just within the hospital. The reported incidence of adverse events during IHT varies from 3% to 75%.[20] Variations of adverse events are due to different definitions, equipment issues, poor documentation of pretransport variables and post-transport management changes. The interhospital transport process largely is unstudied in the United States and demonstrates practices and requirements that vary widely without standardization. Furthermore, multiple handoffs may occur during transport, which increases the risk for communication errors, as shown by many studies. Handoff templates and processes are not standardized for IHTs and only now are becoming standardized for intrahospital transfers due to more available evidence. Despite these challenges, the benefit of IHT must outweigh the risks. Knight and colleagues[21] published a comprehensive review of complications, risk reduction, and prevention during intrahospital transfers in critically ill patients, as illustrated in **Box 1**. Although transferring a sick rural patient to a tertiary center is more complicated, the risks and prevention seem similar to transferring the patient within the hospital.

Pulmonary Complications

For 77 pediatric and neonatal patients, a postintubation chest radiograph recognized that the endotracheal tube was malpositioned in 47% of cases, illustrating the importance of airway position in this population.[22] Of 262 mechanically ventilated adult patients who underwent intrahospital transfer, the 120 adverse events included 0.4% accidental intubation, 8.8% oxygen desaturation, and 17.6% incidents involving

Box 1
Potential risk factors for complications during intrahospital transfer

Patient-related factors

PEEP greater than 6 cm H_2O

History of coronary artery disease

Postoperative patients

Multiple/complex medication/infusion regimens

Increased injury severity (trauma patient)

Facility factors

Distance between the unit of origin and destination

Staff-related factors

Manual ventilation

Treatment modification for transport

Inexperienced staff

Unfamiliarity with equipment/inability to troubleshoot

Insufficient staff education/preparation

Failure to inspect equipment prior to transport

Lack of checklists

Poor communication (within and between departments/units)

Potential risk factors leading to complications during intrahospital transfer are listed according to patient and staff related factors.*Abbreviation:* PEEP, positive end-expiratory pressure.

From Knight PH, Maheshwari N, Hussain J, et al. Complications during intrahospital transport of critically ill patients: focus on risk identification and prevention. Int J Crit Illn Inj Sci. 2015;5(4):256-64; with permission.

airway-related equipment issues. Positive end-expiratory pressure (PEEP) of greater than 6 cm H_2O and treatment modifications prior to transport were associated with increased risk of oxygen desaturation, as reported by Parmentier-Decrucq and colleagues.[23] Most adverse events were equipment-related incidents, including battery issues and alarm settings. Braman and colleagues[24] demonstrated that patients transported by mechanical as opposed to manual ventilation experienced fewer changes in parameters.

Transporting Critically Injured Patients

Patients with spinal, brain, and orthopedic injuries may experience exacerbation of their injuries during the transfer process. Transport by air often involves tight spaces and loud noise, making recurrent assessments challenging. Also, these patients may require multiple episodes of repositioning during the transport. A review of mainly planned intrahospital transports of 288 brain-injured patients with a mean transport time of only 31 minutes resulted in 36% of patients experiencing complications including intracranial hypertension, oxygen desaturation, hypertension or hypotension requiring intervention, and ventilator dyssynchrony.[25] Brain-injured patients with higher injury severity scores are at greater risk of secondary injury during transport, which may be reduced by adequate resuscitation prior to transport. Logic dictates these risks may be compounded by longer interhospital transports, but outcome data are scarce.

Hemodynamic Complications

Postoperative patients and patients with coronary artery disease are more vulnerable to hemodynamic instability and/or arrhythmias. Also, patients on vasopressor support are vulnerable to hemodynamic instability and acid/base disorders. The incidence of cardiac arrest in intrahospital transports is between 0.34% and 1.6%. More than 40% of Medicare beneficiaries who present with acute myocardial infarction, however, are transferred to facilities with revascularization capabilities, which may increase the incidence of cardiac arrest during transport.[26]

Equipment Issues

Specialized retrieval teams are on the rise in Europe. These teams also are trained to problem solve equipment failures. Droogh and colleagues[27] from the Netherlands reviewed the interhospital transports by a ground mobile ICU of 353 critically ill patients and found 55 technical problems over 30 months. The number of technical problems decreased from 26% the first 10 months to 11% during the last 10 months of the study. Technical problems included gas supply issues, electrical issues, ambulance dysfunction, defective battery of ventilators and defibrillators, and trolley dysfunction.[27] Bourn and colleagues[28] from Scotland described setting the standards for IHT, including transfer personnel competencies, as established by the Royal College of Anaesthetists, Faculty of Intensive Care Medicine, and Royal College of Emergency Medicine curricula. Checklists via handheld apps would help to ensure equipment is functioning and information is conveyed.

Interhospital Transfer: Handoffs and Outcomes

Documentation is far from standardized throughout the transfer process and handoffs also are not standardized. Does poor communication harm patients? A change in condition before or during transport is essential information. Does the patient now require pressors or is the patient in respiratory compromise? A retrospective, observational study by Usher and colleagues[29] looked at 335 consecutive patient transfers to 3 ICUs (medical, surgical, and cardiac) at a tertiary academic medical center with the goal of determining what components of the handoff process predicted mortality and adverse outcomes. Records were considered complete with the following:

- Discharge summary
- History and physical examination
- Laboratory values
- Images
- Consults
- Medication reconciliation
- Progress notes

Completeness of documentation was found in only 58.3% of transfers, adverse events occurring within 24 hours of arrival were 42%, and in-hospital mortality was 17.3%. Higher documentation completeness was associated with decreased in-hospital mortality, reduced adverse events, and decreased duplication of labor. The study also noted that documentation volume did not correlate with information content, so a 300-page fax is not helpful. Initiation of transfers began to peak at 8:00 AM, but transfer arrivals peaked during evening and nighttime hours—a time of physician transition. The condition of a critical patient can dramatically change during the 12-hour gap between initiating transfer and arrival. All transfers in this study were coordinated through a transfer center.

Some academic centers are designating a physician coordinator to evaluate incoming transfers in a mini ICU setting as a means of local triage. Although this model still is unstudied, it may help to avoid under-triage or over-triage within the accepting hospital.

The lack of interoperability of electronic health records is yet another barrier in communication. Usher and colleagues[30] noted discordance in comorbidities in more than 85% of IHTs, and 73% of transfers gained a diagnosis whereas 47% lost a diagnosis when looking at more than 130,000 transfers. The study also found a significant reduction in discordance in the 5027 transfers between hospitals participating in a health information exchange. That reduction was not noted in individual participation in a health information exchange.[30]

REVERSE HANDOFF: TRANSITION OF CARE TO HOME

Eventually, rural patients are discharged from the tertiary hospital to return home. The tertiary center often is unfamiliar with the resources and physicians in the rural community. Also, this handoff of transitioning care to home is not standardized. These patients often are transferred due to their high acuity and complexity, but the journey home can be challenging due to poor or even no communication. Although medical record completeness is expected in the IHT process, it often is void in the discharge process. Patients may return home empty handed without records or imaging studies after a prolonged hospitalization. For instance, discharging a patient with a developing 19-cm pancreatic pseudocyst and temporary biliary stent without a handoff is at risk to result in ED visits and readmissions at home.

THE COST OF INTERHOSPITAL TRANSPORT

Interhospital transport is provided by a diversity of organizations, ranging from the local fire department to hospitals to nonprofit organizations to for-profit organizations. Transport occurs by ground or by air. Air transports include fixed-wing or rotary aircraft. Means of transport often are determined by the severity of illness or injury or by distance and geography. The number of air ambulance bases has tripled since a cost assessment more than 20 years ago, giving rural patients access to tertiary care. The actual cost of this service from an operational or pricing standpoint is replete in the literature. Moreover, the calculated costs are different from the price to the patient.

Ground Ambulance

Mulcahy and colleagues[31] in a Medicare Ambulance Services Special Analysis, from July 2019, acknowledged that few data exist of the relationship of Medicare payments and cost of ground ambulance transport. Interhospital transport is covered by Medicare Part A. The urban median ambulance cost per trip of $2000 to $2500 was noted to be significantly higher than the rural median ambulance cost per trip of $1500 despite mile rate charges. The National Registry of Emergency Medical Technicians totaled 387,502 EMS personnel in 2018, with only 100,752 working as paramedics. In rural areas, 75% of the EMS workforce is composed of volunteers compared with only 7.5% in urban areas.[31]

Air Ambulance Cost

According to the Medicare Payment Advisory Commission, in 2011 the average claim for air ambulance was $4908, and the average ground ambulance claim was $322.[32] The median cost per air transport was $10,099, according to an Air Medical Services Cost Study Report.[33] Air transport services used different cost accounting methods, however, thereby limiting this analysis. Approximately 75% of Medicare transports were designated as rural. Median revenue per transport ranged from $354 for self-pay to $23,518 for commercial insurance. Medicare reimbursements covered 59% of costs whereas commercial reimbursements covered 231% of costs. Medicare, Medicaid, commercial, and self-pay made up 37%, 24%, 26%, and 10% of payer mix, respectively.[33] Similar payer mix was reported in a US Government Accountability Office report (GAO-17-637), published in July 2017.[34] **Fig. 2** demonstrates the payer mix of selected providers and range of average payments per transport in 2016.

Financial Risk to Patients

A report by the US Government Accountability Office,[35] from March 2019, reported that 69% of 20,700 studied air transports for privately insured patients were out of network in 2017. Also, between 2010 and 2014 median prices for helicopter transports approximately doubled whereas the number of air ambulance transports increased by 10%. The reports also stated that the median price was $36,400 for a helicopter transport and $40,600 for fixed-wing transport.[35] **Fig. 3** shows the median price change from 2010 to 2014, illustrating a 76% increase according to data from private health insurance compared with the Consumer Price Index increase of 8.5% over the same period, as reported in GAO-17-637.[34] Balance billing privately insured patients may place them at financial risk, because most air transport services do not contract

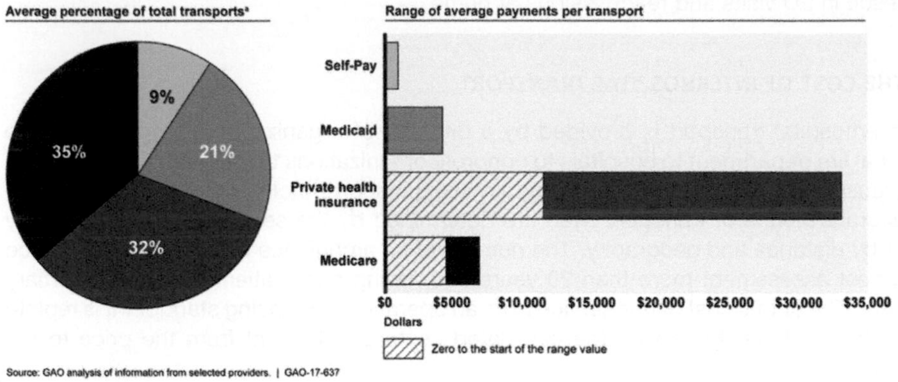

Fig. 2. (*Left*) Average percentage of payer mix of 8 selected air ambulance carriers excluding small "other" category in 2016. (*Right*) Range of average payments per transport in 2016. Note: the 8 selected providers were chosen to represent a range of business model types, sizes, and known perspectives in the industry and included 3 large independent providers and 5 hospital-affiliated providers. [a] Percentages do not add to 100 primarily because they are percentages averaged across the 8 selected providers and because some providers reported percentages that included a small "other" category, which is excluded, containing payers, such as auto or military-sponsored insurance. (*From* United States Government Accountability Office. Report to the committee on transportation and infrastructure, house of representatives. Air ambulance: data collection and transparency needed to enhance DOT oversight. GAO-17-637. Published July 27, 2017. Accessed June 15, 2020. https://www.gao.gov/products/GAO-17-637; with permission.)

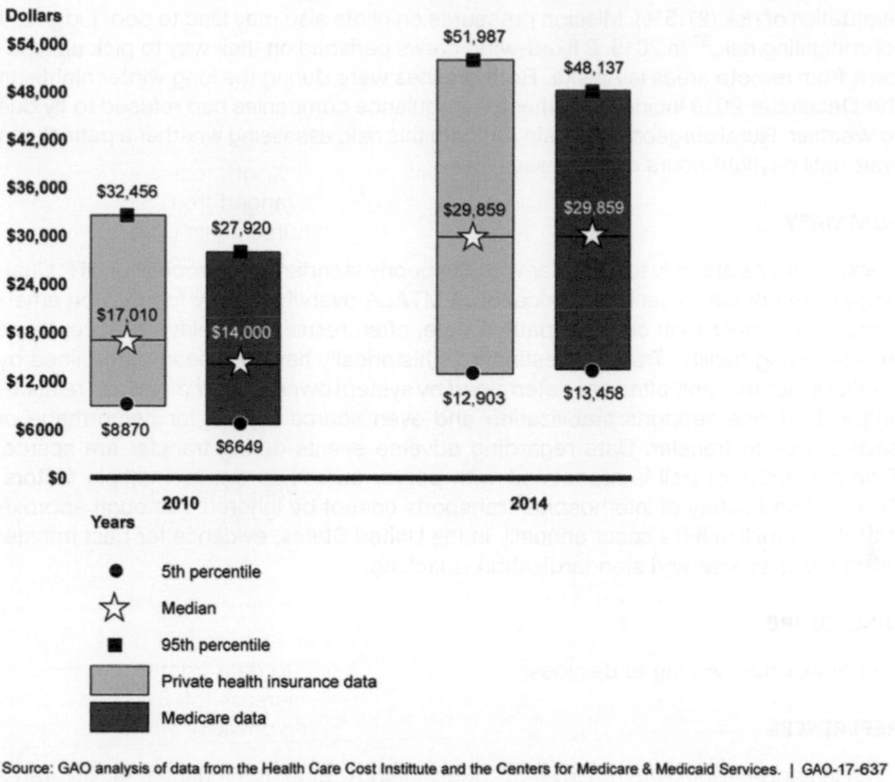

Fig. 3. Median and percentile prices charged for air ambulance service for analyzed Medicare and private health insurance data in 2010 and 2014. Notes: private health insurance data from Health Care Cost Institute may not reflect amounts for all private sector payers. Percentiles indicate the percentage of prices charged that are below the stated amount; for example, 95% of prices charged fall below the 95th percentile. (*From* United States Government Accountability Office. Report to the committee on transportation and infrastructure, house of representatives. Air ambulance: data collection and transparency needed to enhance DOT oversight. GAO-17-637. Published July 27, 2017. Accessed June 15, 2020. https://www.gao.gov/products/GAO-17-637; with permission.)

with private insurance. Contracted payments by private insurers, however, historically have been considered proprietary, leaving patients in the dark about their insurance plan network and coverage.

SAFETY OF TRANSPORT

Many factors weigh in when considering interhospital transport. Safety of the crew and patient, however, is of paramount priority. Because fatalities are more likely to result from crashes in air transport rather than ground transport, the safety of air transport has come under scrutiny. No study directly compares the safety of air versus ground transport, but, from 1992 to 2001, approximately 4500 ground ambulance accidents resulted in 29 fatalities (0.64%). In contrast, from 1998 to 2008, a reported 146 helicopter crashes resulted in 50 fatalities (34%).[36] The most common causes of helicopter air ambulance accidents were mechanical failures (22.5%), controlled flight into terrain often in poor visibility or at night (27.5%), and aeronautic decision making and situation awareness—meaning a pilot's knowledge of factors affecting safety and evaluation of risk (27.5%). Mission pressures on pilots also may lead to poor judgment for mitigating risk.[37] In 2019, 2 fixed-wing crews perished on their way to pick up a patient from remote areas in Alaska. Both crashes were during the long winter nights. In the December 2019 incident, 2 other air ambulance companies had refused to fly due to weather. Rural surgeons can help mitigate this risk, assessing whether a patient can wait until daylight hours or better weather.

SUMMARY

Rural surgeons are only too familiar with the poorly standardized process of IHT. Challenges are unique to each rural location. EMTALA overwhelmingly focuses on emergency care rather than critical inpatient care, often resulting in delays in acceptance at a receiving facility. Transfer destinations historically have not been determined by quality indicators and often are determined by system ownership or physician relationships. Evidence supports stabilization and even source control for hemorrhage or sepsis prior to transfer. Data regarding adverse events during transfer are scarce. Transfer status overall is associated with poorer outcomes due to multiple factors. The cost and safety of interhospital transports cannot be ignored. Although approximately 1.5 million IHTs occur annually in the United States, evidence for best transfer practices is sparse and standardization is lacking.

DISCLOSURE

The author has nothing to disclose.

REFERENCES

1. Hernandez-Boussard T, Davies S, McDonald K, et al. Interhospital facility transfers in the united states: A nationwide outcomes study. J Patient Saf 2017; 13(40):187–91.
2. Bennett K, Probst J, Bullard J, et al. The importance of rural hospitals: Transfers and 30-day readmissions among rural residents and patients presenting at rural hospitals. Popul Health Manag 2019;22(2):120–6.
3. Nguyen YL, Kahn J, Angus D. Reorganizing adult critical delivery: The role of regionalization, telemedicine, and community outreach. Am J Respir Crit Care Med 2010;181:1164–9.
4. Centers for Medicare and Medicaid Services. Medical Learning Network. summary of policies in the calendar year (cy) 2018 medicare physician fee schedule (mpfs) final rule, telehealth originating site facility fee payment amount and telehealth services list, and ct modifier reduction list. 2018. Available at: https://www.cms.gov/Outreach-and-Education/Medicare-Learning-Network-MLN/MLNMattersArticles/downloads/MM10393.pdf. Accessed January 26, 2020.
5. Bosk E, Veinot T, Iwashyna T, et al. Which patients and where: A qualitative study of patient transfers from community hospitals. Med Care 2011;49(6):592–8.
6. Ercan E. Iscan, EMTALA's Oft-Overlooked "Reverse Dumping" Provision and the Implications for Transferee Hospital Liability Following St. Anthony Hospital, 82 WASH. U. L. Q. 1201. 2004. Available at: https://openscholarship.wustl.edu/law_lawreview/vol82/iss3/9. Accessed January 26, 2020.
7. Rush B, Tyler P, Stone D, et al. Outcomes of ventilated patients with sepsis who undergo interhospital transfer. Crit Care Med 2018;46(1):e81–6.
8. Arthur K, Kelz R, Mills A, et al. Interhospital transfer: An independent risk factor for mortality in the surgical intensive care unit. Am Surg 2013;79(9):909–13.

9. Limmer A, Edye M. Interhospital Transfer delays abdominal surgery and prolongs stay. ANZ J Surg 2017;87:867–72.
10. Desai S, Patel J, Abdo H, et al. A comparison of surgical delays in directly admitted versus transferred patients with hip fractures: Opportunities for improvement? Can J Surg 2014;57(1):40–3.
11. Misercola B, Sihler K, Douglas M, et al. Transfer of acute care surgery patients in a rural state: A concerning trend. J Surg Res 2016;206(1):168–74.
12. Sternberg S. Hospitals move to limit low-volume surgeries. Washington, DC: U.S. News and World Report; 2015.
13. Lucas D, Ejaz A, Haut E, et al. Interhospital transfer adverse outcomes after general surgery: Implications for pay for performance. J Am Coll Surg 2014;218(3): 393–400.
14. Crippen C, Hughes S, Chen S, et al. The impact of interhospital transfers on surgical quality metrics for academic medical centers. Am Surg 2014;80(7):690–5.
15. Holcomb J, Helling T, Hirschberg A. Military, civilian, and rural application of the damage control philosophy. Mil Med 2001;166(6):490–3.
16. Harwell P, Reyes J, Helmer S, et al. Outcomes of rural trauma patients who undergo damage control laparotomy. Am J Surg 2019;281(3):490–5.
17. Harvin J, Podbielski J, Vincent L, et al. Damage control laparotomy trial: Design, rationale, and implementation of a randomized controlled trial. Trauma Surg Acute Care Open 2017;2(1):e000083.
18. Waddell G, Scott P, Lees N, et al. Effects of ambulance transport in critically ill patients. BMJ 1975;1:386–9.
19. Waydhas C. Intrahospital transports of critically ill patients. Crit Care 1999;3: R83–9.
20. Droogh J, Smit M, Absalom A, et al. Transferring the critically ill: are we there yet? Cri Care 2015;19(1):62.
21. Knight P, Maheshwari N, Hussain J, et al. Complications during hospital transport of critically ill patients: Focus on identification and prevention. Int J Crit Illn Inj Sci 2015;5(4):256–64.
22. Sanchez-Pinto N, Giuliano J, Schwartz H, et al. The impact of postintubation chest radiograph during pediatric and neonatal critical care transport. Pediatr Crit Care Med 2013;14(5):e213–7.
23. Parmentler-Decrucq E, Poissy J, Nseir S, et al. Adverse events during intrahosptital transport of critically ill patients: Incidence and risk factors. Ann Intensive Care 2013;3(1):10.
24. Braman S, Dunn S, Amico C, et al. Complications of intrahospital transport in critically ill patients. Ann Intern Med 1987;107:468–73.
25. Picetti E, Antonini A, Lucchetti M, et al. Intra-hospital transport of brain-injured patients: A prospective observational study. Neurocrit Care 2013;18:298–304.
26. Iwashyna T, Kayn J, Hayward R, et al. Interhospital transfers among Medicare beneficiaries admitted for acute myocardial infarction at non-revascularization hospitals. Circ Cardiovasc Qual Outcomes 2010;3(5):468–75.
27. Droogh J, Smit M, Hut J, et al. Inter-hosptial Transport of critically ill patients: expect surprises. Crit Care 2012;16(1):R26.
28. Bourn S, Wijesingha S, Nordmann G. Transfer of the critically ill patient. BJA Education 2018;18(3):63–8.
29. Usher M, Fanning C, Wu D, et al. Information handoff and outcomes of critically ill patients transferred between hospitals. J Crit Care 2016;36:240–5.

30. Usher M, Sahni N, Herrigel D, et al. Diagnostic discordance, Health Information Exchange, and inter-hospital transfer outcomes: A population study. J Gen Intern Med 2018;33:1447–53.
31. Mulcahy A, Becker K, Cantor J, et al. Medicare's ground ambulance data collection system: sampling and instrument considerations and recommendations. Centers for Medicare & Medicaid Services; 2019. Available at: https://www.cms.gov/Medicare/Medicare-Fee-for-Service-Payment/AmbulanceFeeSchedule/Downloads/Ground-Ambulance-Data-Collection-System-Sampling-Instrument-Considerations-Recommendations.pdf. Accessed January 26, 2020.
32. Medicare Payment Advisory Commission (MedPAC). June 2013 Report to Congress, Chapter 7: Mandated report: Medicare payment for ambulance services. Available at: http://www.medpac.gov/docs/default-source/reports/jun13_ch07_appendix.pdf?sfvrsn=0. Accessed January 26, 2020.
33. Air Medical Services Cost Study Report. Xcenda AmerisourceBergen. 2017. Available at: https://aams.org/wp-content/uploads/2017/04/Air-Medical-Services-Cost-Study-Report.pdf. Accessed January 26, 2020.
34. Unites States Government Accountability Office (GAO-17-637). Air Ambulance: Data Collection and Transparency Needed to Enhance DOT Oversight. 2017. Available at: https://www.gao.gov/assets/690/686167.pdf. Accessed January 27, 2020.
35. United States Government Accountability Office (GAO-19-292). Air Ambulance: Available Data Show Privately-Insured Patients are at Financial Risk. 2019. Available at: https://www.gao.gov/assets/700/697684.pdf. Accessed January 26, 2020.
36. Steenhoff TC, Zohn SF. EMS, Air Medical Transport. In: StatPearls. Treasure Island (FL): StatPearls Publishing; 2020. Available at: https://www.ncbi.nlm.nih.gov/books/NBK482358/. Accessed January 26, 2020.
37. Elias B. Congressional research service for congress. Safety of air ambulances 2006. Available at: https://www.everycrsreport.com/files/20060523_RL33430_90eddbcb5ea4581c169d46a88c53882b11d3c831.pdf. Accessed January 26, 2020.

Regionalization of General Surgery Within the Mayo Clinic Health System and the Mayo Clinic

Michael Roskos, MD[a,b,*], Megan Nelson, MD[c,d]

KEYWORDS

• Regionalization • Surgery • Volume • Outcomes • Robotics • Mayo • Patient • Locums

KEY POINTS

- The Mayo Clinic is actively engaged in regionalization of surgery within its health system. It has embraced a nonvolume outcome approach. Unexpected outcomes are expeditiously reviewed facilitating process improvement and improved care.
- Patients often make the counterintuitive decision to receive their care locally despite poorer outcomes. These decisions have been driven by patient factors, such as transportation, life disruption, finances, poor health, and remoteness.
- The Mayo Clinic Health system compares favorably to Mayo Clinic Rochester with surgical outcomes in the more common surgeries, which make up almost 40% of the individual health system surgical volumes.
- The Mayo Clinic has made it a priority to train Health System surgeons in new procedures and advanced technology facilitating surgical care closer to home for patients.
- Implementing surgical regionalization is supported but poorly described. The Mayo Clinic has many examples of regionalization implemented in the health system. This includes hybrid surgeon positions, Mayo-specific locums, and back referrals from Mayo Rochester to the Health System sites. Overcoming patient barriers is an important part of regionalization.

[a] Department of General Surgery, Mayo Clinic La Crosse Fransican Healthcare, 700 West Avenue South, La Crosse, WI 54601, USA; [b] Rural Track General Surgery Residency Program, Mayo Clinic Integrated Community and Rural Surgery, Mayo Clinic, Rochester, MN, USA; [c] Division of Community General Surgery, Mayo Clinic, 1216 Second Street Southwest, Rochester, MN 55902, USA; [d] Department of Trauma, Critical Care and General Surgery, Mayo Clinic, Rochester, MN, USA

* Corresponding author. Department of General Surgery, Mayo Clinic La Crosse Franciscan Healthcare, Mayo Clinic, 700 West Avenue South, La Crosse, WI 54601.
E-mail address: Roskos.Michael@mayo.edu

Surg Clin N Am 100 (2020) 937–948
https://doi.org/10.1016/j.suc.2020.07.002 surgical.theclinics.com

OBJECTIVE

This article describes regionalization of general surgery within the Mayo Clinic Health System and the Mayo Clinic in Rochester.

INTRODUCTION

Regionalization of general surgery refers to the concentration of complex or low-volume surgeries at a smaller number of regional centers. This concept has been supported by the inverse relationship of surgical volume and mortalities demonstrated in the work of Luft[1] and Birkmeyer and colleagues.[2,3] Increased hospital volume is often correlated with lower complication rates, lower reoperation rates, lower admission rates, lower mortalities, and lower costs.[4] Currently, volume-related outcomes form the basis for the Volume Pledge[5] and the Leapfrog Group recommendations,[6] both of which are strong advocates of surgical regionalization.

Despite the appeal for regionalization of high-risk procedures, they still commonly take place in low-volume centers.[7] Potentially even more alarming is that few hospitals meet the "take the pledge" volume thresholds.[8]

Although the merits of volume-based regionalization may support its implementation, many competing factors continue to prevent fully embracing implementation of the concept. At the heart of these factors are those concerning to patients. Symer and colleagues[9] included in their study 6 major qualitative themes when describing patient-related barriers. These barriers included transportation, life disruption, tangible social support, socioeconomic barriers, poor health, and remoteness.

Further complicating implementation may be the patients' reluctance to travel despite higher, oftentimes much higher, mortalities. In a seminal 1999 study, Finlayson and colleagues[10] demonstrated that patients preferred local surgery despite a decidedly higher local surgical mortality (**Table 1**).

Resio and colleagues[11] showed that superior outcomes were powerful motivators for some patients to travel to regional high-volume sites for surgery. For the remaining patients, the most important facilitator (factor?) to travel to a regional center was addressing the challenges of travel, such as transportation, parking, and housing. Understanding and implementing successful regionalization mean balancing the patients' needs and the patients' wants.

Some may find it surprising that a surgical center's reputation and outcomes might not automatically be the deciding factor in whether patients can or will choose that facility, be it a high-risk, low-volume surgery or low-risk, high-volume one. One reason

Table 1
Mortality preferences

Local Mortality, %	Preference to Stay Local, %
6	45
12	23
18	18

Regional mortality = 3%.

Data from Finlayson SRG, Birkmeyer JD, Tosteson ANA, et al. Patient preferences for location of care - Implications for regionalization. *Med Care.* 1999;37(2):204-209.

there is increasing pressure placed on local providers to provide local care. These complexities of choice, along with other factors, play a role in the reluctance of some institutions to describe their implementation of regionalization. Mayo Enterprise has embraced nonvolume-related outcomes via their multidisciplinary approach to quality, which includes electronic health record data mining, use of risk-adjusted registries, such as the National Surgical Quality Improvement Program (NSQIP), and internal performance improvement processes.[4] No mandates exist, and Mayo Clinic in Rochester (Rochester) offers consultations and even multidisciplinary reviews. High-risk, low-volume surgeries make up only a small portion of surgeries at smaller centers. Losing this care is not likely to influence finances.[12] Concentrating resources on regional surgery whereby 40% of surgeries consist of 5 types can make for a different kind of regionalization, one that supports advanced training and technology and provides outcomes data to the smaller community that may be focusing on quality and financial implications. Developing services related to 5 high-volume surgeries is far more manageable than trying to do the same for 228 procedures, as described in the literature discussing the heterogeneity of general surgery.[13]

By describing regionalization within the Mayo Clinic Health System, the authors add to a growing body of knowledge regarding the regionalization of general surgery that has potential applications in all surgical practices and health systems, regardless of their size and scope of practice.

BACKGROUND

Mayo Clinic, the enterprise, includes major campuses in Minnesota, Arizona, and Florida and provides care to more than 1 million people per year. Institutionally, Mayo Clinic has a history of quality outcome reporting.[14] Mayo Clinic has intermittently participated in the volume-focused Leapfrog hospital survey. Although meeting "The Volume Pledge" volume thresholds, Mayo Clinic has not joined this initiative until recently because it was thought it would not significantly impact its practices as a quality-minded, high-volume center. Mayo Clinic continues to focus on outcome quality managed at the facility level.[4]

Mayo Clinic has facilities in rural communities, which make up the Mayo Clinic Health System. It is located in 4 geographically divided areas, based on hub sites that surround Rochester in western Wisconsin, eastern Minnesota, and northeast Iowa. The Mayo Clinic Health System serves 60 communities with 1000 providers and 42 general surgeons. The general surgeon's scope of practice in the Mayo Clinic Health System has included everything from complex aortic repairs to colonoscopies and C-sections. The hubs in La Crosse, Wisconsin; Eau Claire, Wisconsin; Mankato, Minnesota; and Rochester, Minnesota serve as higher-level care centers for many of the rural clinics and critical care access hospitals within their geographic areas. The hub sites in La Crosse, Eau Claire, and Mankato also refer to the Mayo Clinic in Rochester. The hubs are representative of a general surgery practice, as indicated by the top 5 surgeries performed at each hub site (**Table 2**). The Mayo Clinic Health System hires its general surgeons, which are employees of Mayo Clinic, but may operate in non-Mayo Clinic–owned hospitals. Historically, the Mayo Clinic Health System, specifically, each hub site, hired its own general surgeons. Currently, all Health System general surgeons are vetted, interviewed, and hired by Rochester Mayo. Mayo Clinic Health System general surgeons are under the quality oversight of both local and Rochester-based quality assessment teams.

Mayo Clinic Health System's La Crosse campus (MCHS–La Crosse) is representative of the other hub sites, and we consider ourselves sensitive to the issues of rural

Table 2
Top 5 general surgery cases at hub sites 2018

Hub Site	Eau Claire	Mankato	Austin/Albert Lea[a]	La Crosse
1	Laparoscopic cholecystectomy with cholangiogram	Laparoscopic cholecystectomy	Laparoscopic cholecystectomy	Placement port-a-cath - power port
2	Repair hernia inguinal with mesh	Laparoscopic appendectomy	Laparoscopic appendectomy	Laparoscopic cholecystectomy with cholangiogram
3	Laparoscopic appendectomy	Repair hernia inguinal with mesh	Repair hernia inguinal with mesh	Laparoscopic cholecystectomy
4	Laparoscopic cholecystectomy	Placement port-a-cath power port	Laparoscopic cholecystectomy with cholangiogram	Laparoscopic appendectomy
5	Repair hernia umbilical with mesh	Repair ventral hernia with mesh	Laparoscopic hernia repair–inguinal extraperitoneal	Laparoscopic hernia repair–inguinal–transabdominal
Total				
Percentage of total cases at site	35	42	44	36

Colonoscopies are the most common procedure.
[a] Technically Rochester is the hub site, but Austin/Albert Lea represent the community practice.
Unpublished data, Courtesy of the Mayo Clinic, Rochester, MN.

surgery; although we work in a county of around 115,000 residents, we still perform surgeries that range from endoscopy to complex lung cases. Outcomes of the most common surgeries compare favorably with Rochester, which correlate with the previous work of Ibrahim and colleagues[15] (**Table 3**).

Those included on the Leapfrog table (**Table 4**) make up a minority of the La Crosse cases. Notable exceptions include carotid endarterectomies and lung resections for cancer. La Crosse does not have a carotid stenting program despite a robust Rochester-based effort to develop one. It was agreed by La Crosse general surgeons that carotid stenting volume could not justify the program. Aortic surgical outcomes resulted in referrals for aortic surgery to Mayo Clinic in Rochester, where open and endovascular aortic surgery could be reliably offered. Of note, a competing local hospital, nearly twice our size and less than 1 mile away from the La Crosse campus, has a vascular center, a carotid stenting program, aortic endovascular capabilities, and cardiothoracic surgeons. This hospital is also a level II trauma center (Mayo La Crosse is level III trauma center) with 2 helicopters. It gives local patients an alternative to driving 70 miles to Rochester.

We also work with rural surgeons within our health system, provide outreach services to these sites, and have hired rural surgeons within our system. In addition, La Crosse has been influential in developing the rural track residency program based in Rochester.[16] Our breadth of practice in La Crosse is fertile ground for a broad-

Table 3
Mayo Hub Site Variation based on 2018 National Surgical Quality Improvement Program data

Procedure	Range/Actual Hub Site
Laparoscopic cholecystectomy no intraoperative cholangiogram (IOC) as a % of all laparoscopic cholecystectomy (with and without intraoperative cholangiogram)	2%–88% (2%, 4%, 52%, 88%)
Laparoscopic inguinal hernia repair as a % of all inguinal hernia repairs (open + laparoscopic)	7%–67% (7%, 29%, 31%, 67%)
Laparoscopic colectomy as a % of all colectomies (open + laparoscopic)	29%–56%, (29%, 48%, 56%, 56%)
Open colectomy SSI	8%–20% (8%, 9%, 15%, 20%)
Laparoscopic colectomy length of stay	3.7–6.6 d (3.7, 4.2, 6.4, 6.6)
Open colectomy length of stay	7.6–9.6 d (7.6, 8.7, 8.9, 9.6)
Expected morbidity open colectomy	0.026–0.193 (0.026, 0.189, 0.193, 0.193)

Data from American College of Surgeons National Surgical Quality Improvement Program, 2019, ACS NSQIP Semiannual Report July 12, 2019. Chicago: American College of Surgeons.

based general surgical practice and rural track resident training. Our experience is special, as is the case with other Mayo Clinic Health System hub sites, in that we must decide each day which surgeon should be doing which surgery at which location, both as a receiving hospital and as a referring hospital to Rochester.

REGIONALIZATION

Regionalization and the discussion of regionalization have mostly revolved around low-volume procedures. However, it has become increasingly clear that

Table 4
Leapfrog and volume pledge procedure lists

Leapfrog, s/h	Volume Pledge, s/h
Bariatric, 20/50	Bariatric, 20/40
Esophageal resection for cancer, 7/20	Esophageal resection for cancer, 5/20
Lung resection for cancer, 15/40	Lung resection for cancer, 20/40
Pancreatic resection for cancer, 10/20	Pancreatic resection for cancer, 5/20
Rectal cancer, 6/16	Rectal cancer, 6/15
Carotid endarterectomy, 10/20	Carotid stenting, 5/10
Open aortic surgeries, 7/10	Complex aortic surgery, 8/20
Mitral valve replacement, 20/40	Mitral valve repair, 10/20
	Hip replacement, 25/50
	Knee replacement, 25/50

Abbreviations: h, hospital minimum; s, surgeon minimum.

Data from Leapfrog. Surgical Volume. The Leapfrog Group Web site. https://www.leapfroggroup.org/ratings-reports/surgical-volume. Updated n.d. Accessed 25 February 2020; and Urbach DR. Pledging to Eliminate Low-Volume Surgery. *New Engl J Med.* 2015;373(15):1388-1390.

regionalization could just as well apply to high-volume procedures or could also mean supporting surgery in the region. In the past, this might have been understood as regional smaller centers (such as Mayo Clinic Health System hospitals) referring surgeries to Mayo Clinic in Rochester. More recent regionalization practices could be seen as supporting regional surgical practice by discussing surgeries, accepting challenging patients in transfer, or providing resource-based oncology care requiring a multidisciplinary approach.

EARLY REGIONALIZATION

Early regionalization was largely based on individual surgeons making individual decisions about which surgeries were done where. This early regionalization was based on the individual surgeon's training and comfort level balanced with patient's choices or preferences. At MCHS–La Crosse, most pancreatic, liver, and esophageal resections, especially if they involved cancer, were referred to Rochester. We continued to operate on abdominal aortic aneurysms, carotids, rectal cancers, and complex lung cancers. Unexpected outcomes were reviewed. Rarely were we prohibited from performing surgeries, based on a single case. As the complexity of oncologic care evolved, almost all sarcoma and a high percentage of rectal cancers are now referred to Rochester.

INTERNAL REGIONALIZATION

Regionalization within Mayo Clinic's sites became more formalized with the concept of One Mayo. Initiated approximately 10 years ago, this initiative strives to offer the same care to every patient, no matter what Mayo Enterprise door the patient walks through. At a high level, One Mayo improved its ability to recruit surgeons through offering hybrid surgeon positions or "surgeon trade," defined site capabilities (facilities designation capabilities), pioneered a Mayo-specific internal locum tenens coverage, and for the first time, facilitated institutional-appropriate surgical patients referrals to Health System sites closer to patients' homes. Perhaps more importantly, Mayo Clinic in Rochester intensified its scrutiny of high-risk/low-volume surgeries and aggressively trained and continues to train Health System surgeons in institutional-appropriate higher-volume surgeries, such as robotic hernia repairs (ventral and inguinal) and gallbladder removal, as well as low-risk procedures such as rib fixation.

Hybrid Surgeon/Surgeon Trade

The facilities within the Mayo Clinic Health System include remote rural communities. The Mayo Clinic surgeon trade strives to maintain skills of low-volume/community/hub site Health System surgeons as well as minimize the referring slippery slope that comes with the deterioration of these skills. This hybrid position has been developed over the last 6 years. The community surgeon rotates into the high-volume facility, such as Rochester, and vice versa for one to 2 weeks as a full-fledged team member providing the care not only with surgery but also with comprehensive preoperative and postoperative care.[4] It allows the community surgeon to manage both the planned and the unexpected complex surgery better. Most importantly, it improves the understanding of the infrastructure necessary to support complex cases. It also helps to determine which cases could be done in the lower-volume locations. In addition, high-volume surgeons spend time in the lower-volume center and experience first-hand the environment and the challenges that come with a lower-volume facility. The high-volume surgeons and centers understand more effective ways to support the community surgical practices. This exchange of surgeons has been critical in helping integrate the community and hub practices within the Health System. It also led to substantial improvement in standardization across all practice sites. In addition, the networking that comes with working with colleagues from different locations results in improved and more collegial communications.

Defined Site Capabilities (Facilities Designation Capabilities)

The Mayo Clinic Health System surgeons conducted the painstaking process of determining capabilities at each surgical site and developed the pyramid of care of general surgery in the Health System. They defined hours of operation for surgical services, on-call coverage, average length of stay, trauma coverage, intensive care unit coverage, quality, patient rescue needs, transfer plans, and procedures guidelines. Community or hub site surgeons had an active role in these definitions, and by doing so conducted an honest and transparent evaluation of surgical facilities and capabilities.

Mayo Clinic–Based Internal Locum Tenens

Invariably, gaps in surgical coverage occur, for any number of reasons. Smaller communities are much more affected by these absences whereby one or 2 surgeons may be covering, but even hub sites feel the effect of a "lost" partner. Patients are temporarily and sometimes permanently diverted to a high-volume center, potentially overwhelming that center. Patients must travel, unexpectedly, for surgeries that could be done closer to home. Non–Mayo locum tenens surgical coverage can be expensive and unpredictable and may lead to variable surgical outcomes. Mayo Clinic in Rochester has a dedicated internal locum tenens surgeon position that, after a 2-year trial, is now a permanent position. This position is vetted, interviewed, and hired by Mayo Rochester, similar to a regular surgical position. The only real difference is an openness to schedule flexibility, allowing for system-wide coverage on an as-needed basis. Not only has this been proven a necessity by the extent of this provider's coverage throughout the health system, but also because this person spends time at both high-volume (Rochester) and low-volume centers within the Mayo Clinic Health System, this person has been insightful regarding the differences between sites. A second Mayo-based internal locum is being trialed with a focus on endoscopy coverage.

Back Referrals

Because the Rochester practice manages challenging access, alternative ways of expedited surgical evaluation and treatment have been developed. Rochester referrals with institutional-appropriate surgical problems are screened, and patients are given the option to obtain their care closer to home in other Mayo Clinic or Health System sites. Surgical wait time has been decreased from months to days as a result, especially for operations such as hernia repair and gallbladder removal.

Increased Scrutiny of Surgical Outcomes

Unexpected surgical outcomes are reviewed, and in some cases, presented in person at Rochester within days of the outcome. In essence, we have an as-needed, *expeditious*, region-wide morbidity and mortality ad hoc meeting completed at either the hub sites or at Rochester. As efforts continue to quickly improve care, the number of these presentations has increased in the last several years and has resulted in improved learning and process improvement, and in rare cases, limiting surgeries allowed at hub sites.

Practice Line Development

Proactive regionalization of surgery has occurred in the Mayo Health System and is viewed favorably as bringing additional surgery options to the Mayo Clinic Health System. This proactive regionalization of surgery has been observed with the initiation of rib fixation in La Crosse in March 2018 and the introduction of robotic general surgery at several sites starting in August 2018. In both cases, Mayo Clinic in Rochester supported the industry training and in-house mentored training in Rochester that emphasized efforts to bring those surgeries to the health system safely and closer to patients who would benefit from them.

Robotics

At Mayo Clinic in Rochester, robotics is considered the next step in the evolution of general surgery, similar to the transition from open surgery to laparoscopy. It allows for the precision of surgery to be infinitely refined and improved as the technology improves. Currently, a robot at a hospital is a large financial outlay, but Mayo Clinic recognizes that for common procedures, patients should have the same access to technology and techniques, no matter their location or the time of their presentation. Robotics in the health system is representative of that commitment to access. As a result, robotics training for the community surgeon has taken center stage. Our first general surgery case in the health system was in Mankato in August 2018. Since then, 10 community-based surgeons have been trained. Formal training takes 2 days, but the preparation leading up to it usually occurs over a few months. The 2-day training course at can be done on-site at Mayo Clinic in Rochester, where we participate in simulation laboratory, porcine laboratory, and a surgeon-led cadaver laboratory. This on-site training was a first of its kind and was the culmination of the collaboration of the Mayo Clinic with industry partners. The surgeon must then do 3 to 5 proctored cases at their hospital with an expert robotics surgeon present. Additional training courses are provided when the surgeon would like to add procedures to their robotics arsenal. Usually, the surgeon's home hospital pays for the training. Mayo Clinic–based proctors decrease the training costs considerably. Robotic cases in La Crosse alone have gone from 13 in 2018 to 69 in 2019 (Roskos, 2019, Unpublished data). This number is expected to increase in 2020.

Rib Fixation

Rib fractures are an important part of MCHS–La Crosse's low-volume trauma service. Rib-fracture patients were being transferred to Mayo Clinic in Rochester for both operative and nonoperative treatment. The trauma department at Rochester supported La Crosse's effort to learn the management of rib fractures, including rib fixation. Rochester-based hands-on mentoring was provided for 2 community-based surgeons. The index surgeons also completed industry-supported training. The first rib fixation procedure was completed March 2018. In 2018, of 27 patients with rib fracture, 3 have had rib fixation. In 2019, 49 patients were admitted with rib fractures, and 6 patients had rib fixation. Numerous transfers to Rochester have given way to local care for all rib fracture patients. The surgeons in La Crosse and Rochester remain closely collaborative to optimize patient selection.

Both robotics and the rib-fixation practices have been excellent examples of targeted and careful adoption of new procedures in the health system, with access to ongoing mentoring; this is a model Mayo Clinic will continue to use in the future.

EXTERNAL FACTORS AFFECTING REGIONALIZATION

External factors can also affect the regionalization of surgery. These external factors may include National Comprehensive Cancer Network guidelines, American College of Surgeons trauma center verification, and American College of Surgeons Children's Surgery verification. Most of these requirements balance volume with the financial implications tied to those. Other factors include cancer practices requiring multidisciplinary multimodality treatments, such as intraoperative radiation, specialized staging modalities such as endobronchial ultrasound/endoscopic ultrasound, or readily accessible PET scanners, and board-certified surgical subspecialists' active participation in multidisciplinary patient care discussions, which could only be justified at tertiary or quaternary centers. In La Crosse, teleconferences have provided widely successful multidisciplinary vascular conferences with clear applications in cancer multidisciplinary conferencing; mobile radiology units have also alleviated some of these concerns. Other external factors may include geography (crossing state lines), insurance, local hospital and clinic competitors, and local ambulance/air transport services. All of these play a role in the regionalization of surgery in the Mayo Clinic Health System.

DISCUSSION

There is no doubt that the outcomes of elective surgery are better when an operation is done by a high-volume surgeon in a high-volume hospital.[5] There is also no doubt that surgical outcomes reflect more than volume: good surgical technique and team proficiency, proper support systems, sound hospital processes, and appropriate patient selection are essential.[4] The fact remains, however, that absolute volumes thresholds are arbitrary and do not account for the longitudinal experiences of people, teams, and services[17] as evidenced by the threshold variation in the Pledge and Leapfrog volume requirements (see **Table 4**). Further complicating the overwhelming numbers of published volume studies is confusion surrounding the nuances of the statistical analysis, which makes definitive interpretation challenging and potentially subject to significant bias.[4]

Surgical regionalization remains contentious and difficult to implement. Many high-risk surgeries still occur in low-volume centers.[7] Regionalization has focused on only a few types of low-volume, high-risk surgeries. In many cases, it has focused on referrals, and not keeping patients. The Mayo Clinic understands that regionalization includes making local surgery better and, at times, referring patients back to local facilities. The Mayo Clinic also realizes that patients may not make the decision to travel to high-volume centers because of many patient factors,[17] providing motivation to optimize care in regional centers.

Patient Factors

The needs and potentially the wants of the patient continue to drive surgery regionalization. It is presumed patients want the best care possible, and for many, that is true. However, for regionalization within Mayo Clinic or anywhere else to work, we must understand that patients will sometimes make the counterintuitive decision to receive high-risk procedures at low-volume centers, even at the cost of significantly higher mortalities.[10] Patients' life needs may be as important as their medical needs, and these life needs may be easier for them to understand and manage. Health care providers' understanding of patients' barriers to receiving care from high-volume centers, such as travel costs, is crucial for the development of regionalization system, which encourages patients to commit to receiving their high-risk procedures at a high-volume center. This includes limiting travel barriers in addition to cost, such as transportation choices, other financial burdens, such as missed work or higher care costs at high-volume centers, or patients' fears, founded or unfounded, of the potential added risks when postoperative complications are managed by a hospital closer to home, but not the one performing the surgery. Regionalization within the Mayo Clinic Health System is a delicate balance between outcomes and the financial and emotional burdens to patients.

Nonpatient Factors

Nonpatient factors to be addressed include the hospital and referring physician needs, such as getting patients onto the schedules of high-volume surgeons at high-volume centers. It will be important to focus on transparency of specific surgical limitations. Institutions must be transparent about available procedures and about the outcomes of high-volume surgeons at referral centers. For regionalization to work, local hospitals must be cognizant that referring these surgeries will not have a huge financial impact if transfers are carefully limited to the most complex.[12] In addition, referring low-risk surgeries back to the hub sites eliminates any potential losses, keeps patients closer to home, and takes the load off overwhelmed regional centers.[18] Fragmented care can be deleterious to surgical patients.[19] Processes that both educate the patient regarding the value of regionalization and provide access to the high-volume center as seamlessly and effortlessly as possible are consistent with the One Mayo concept.

There are numerous other nonpatient factors. Adverse outcomes of any type may be scrutinized to the point where surgeons may choose to decrease their practice or avoid certain surgical patients. This would impact an already busy Rochester practice and perhaps allow deterioration of surgical comfort and skills. Leadership must be clear, with minimal redundancy. A unified plan crossing all surgical subspecialties is an ideal, but is not practical. Ideal surgical leaders have valuable insights and work experience at both Rochester and Health System surgical practices and can equally advocate for both. Finally, conflicting agendas that pit surgical outcomes against financial ones must be transparently discussed.

Mayo Clinic will continue to use its multidimensional approach to quality, which includes electronic health record data mining and analysis, use of risk-adjusted registries such as NSQIP, and initial performance improvement processes designed to immediately identify and address quality issues when they occur. Mayo Clinic will once again participate in the Leapfrog hospital survey in 2020 under the strategic direction of Mayo Clinic's new chief executive officer. Mayo Clinic does not plan to join the volume pledge initiative.[4] Unfortunately, participating in NSQIP does not guarantee change.[20]

There are numerous interesting questions resulting from the comparison of Rochester's and hubs sites' NSQIP common surgeries outcomes data, providing fertile ground to discuss differences throughout the Enterprise. Differences might include indications for cholangiograms, variability of open versus laparoscopic inguinal hernia rates, significantly lower-than-expected morbidities in one of the 4 hospitals, and decidedly higher surgical site infection (SSI) rates in open colon patients despite similar average expected morbidity rates. Discussing and analyzing these data can improve care at all sites. Sharing these data makes referrals back to the health system easier to justify as well as making it understandable for the patient. This data may give the enterprise an opportunity to mesh both quality and cost to provide value; this might include the use of magnetic resonance cholangiopancreatographys, endoscopic retrograde cholangiopancreatography, cholangiograms, and various cautery devices and stapling devices.

Such data have limitations. They refer to a surgery, not a specific surgeon and are limited by resources available in some cases. American College of Surgeons-provided risk stratification does not allow direct comparisons to other NSQIP hospitals.

Colonoscopy data clearly confirm that sites share similar cecal intubation rates and adhere to a 6-minute withdrawal time. The adenoma detection rate, considered the preferred quality measure, is available but is in the process of being validated. Confirming universal quality, the question has become where to do the colonoscopies not which physician or department does them, making colonoscopies more accessible and potentially closer to patients' homes.

Telemedicine will likely play a major role in regionalization of surgery. The COVID pandemic has catapulted telemedicine into routine use for new consultations and postoperative visits. It has been largely well received by patients and surgical providers alike. Telemedicine will likely play a role in regionalization of surgical within the Mayo System, not only in patients' care but also more personalized communication among surgical providers.

Mayo Clinic's history of success will be challenged as it continues to negotiate the challenges of surgical regionalization, a process that embraces support of the low-volume center through collegial interactions and practice line development, a concept that more than ever illustrates Mayo Clinic's commitment to quality patient care as close to home as possible.

Helping health system surgeons to feel comfortable in their decisions to operate or transfer will be just as important as it once was. It must be done in the context of a willingness to learn and review outcomes, as well as communicating with colleagues and taking time with the patient. Regionalization may be the best and most honest way to get our patients to the right place, with the right surgeon, at the right time.

ACKNOWLEDGMENTS

The authors thank Heather Jett, MLS, Mayo Clinic Libraries, Sharon Trester, MS, Mayo Clinic Department of Surgery, and Sharon Nehring RN, BSN, Sr Program Manager Research NSQIP Mayo Rochester, for their invaluable assistance with this article.

DISCLOSURE

Dr. Megan Nelson is an instructor and consultant for Intuitive Surgical, has instructed an American Hernia Society course funded by Medtronic, and is a consultant for Allergan.

REFERENCES

1. Luft HS, Bunker JP, Enthoven AC. Should operations be regionalized - empirical relation between surgical volume and mortality. N Engl J Med 1979;301(25):1364–9.
2. Birkmeyer JD, Siewers AE, Finlayson EVA, et al. Hospital volume and surgical mortality in the United States. N Engl J Med 2002;346(15):1128–37.
3. Birkmeyer JD, Stukel TA, Siewers AE, et al. Surgeon volume and operative mortality in the United States. N Engl J Med 2003;349(22):2117–27.
4. Board DH, editor. Low-volume high-risk surgical procedures: surgical volume and its relationship to patient safety and quality of care. Second Report. Falls Church (VA): United States of America Department of Defense; 2019.
5. Urbach DR. Pledging to eliminate low-volume surgery. N Engl J Med 2015;373(15):1388–90.

6. Leapfrog. Surgical volume. The Leapfrog Group Web site. Available at: https://www.leapfroggroup.org/ratings-reports/surgical-volume. Accessed February 25, 2020.
7. Harrison S, Tangel V, Wu X, et al. Are minimum volume standards appropriate for lung and esophageal surgery? J Thorac Cardiovasc Surg 2018;155(6):2683–94.e1.
8. Jacobs RC, Groth S, Farjah F, et al. Potential impact of "take the volume pledge" on access and outcomes for gastrointestinal cancer surgery. Ann Surg 2019;270(6):1079–89.
9. Symer MM, Abelson JS, Yeo HL. Barriers to regionalized surgical care: public perspective survey and geospatial analysis. Ann Surg 2019;269(1):73–8.
10. Finlayson SRG, Birkmeyer JD, Tosteson ANA, et al. Patient preferences for location of care - implications for regionalization. Med Care 1999;37(2):204–9.
11. Resio BJ, Chiu AS, Hoag JR, et al. Motivators, barriers, and facilitators to traveling to the safest hospitals in the United States for complex cancer surgery. Jama Netw Open 2018;1(7):e184595.
12. Chappel AR, Zuckerman RS, Finlayson SRG. Small rural hospitals and high-risk operations: how would regionalization affect surgical volume and hospital revenue? J Am Coll Surg 2006;203(5):599–604.
13. Decker MR, Dodgion CM, Kwok AC, et al. Specialization and the current practices of general surgeons. J Am Coll Surg 2014;218(1):8–15.
14. U.S. News & World Report Best Hospitals Rankings 2019-2020. US News & World Report 2019.
15. Ibrahim AM, Hughes TG, Thumma JR, et al. Association of hospital critical access status with surgical outcomes and expenditures among Medicare beneficiaries. JAMA 2016;315(19):2095–103.
16. Randy C, Lehman M, Brandon G, et al. Mayo Clinic joins the national effort to train tomorrow's rural surgeons. Bull Am Coll Surg 2019;104(10):33–8.
17. Livingston EH, Cao J. Procedure volume as a predictor of surgical outcomes. JAMA 2010;304(1):95–7.
18. Brooke BS, Goodney PP, Kraiss LW, et al. Readmission destination and risk of mortality after major surgery: an observational cohort study. Lancet 2015;386(9996):884–95.
19. Justiniano CF, Xu Z, Becerra AZ, et al. Long-term deleterious impact of surgeon care fragmentation after colorectal surgery on survival: continuity of care continues to count. Dis Colon Rectum 2017;60(11):1147–54.
20. Osborne NH, Nicholas LH, Ryan AM, et al. Association of hospital participation in a quality reporting program with surgical outcomes and expenditures for Medicare beneficiaries. JAMA 2015;313(5):496–504.

Using Qualitative Research to Study the Profession of Rural Surgery

Dorothy Hughes, MHSA, PhD[a,b,*], Joanna Veazey Brooks, MBE, PhD[a]

KEYWORDS

• Rural surgery • Qualitative research • Systematic review

KEY POINTS

- Qualitative studies about rural surgery in the last 10 years have primarily used interviews and focus groups to explore questions about patient experiences.
- Obstetrics is a specialty frequently explored in qualitative rural surgery studies, and the provision of rural surgical services is a frequent topic of investigation.
- Data collection methods, such as participant observation and ethnography, could gather qualitative data critical to better understanding the social context of rural surgery.
- Qualitative methods could be used in future rural surgery research to address surgical teamwork, scope of practice, workforce, and the aging rural patient population.

INTRODUCTION

The objective of this article was to systematically review existing, peer-reviewed literature to understand the breadth and depth of qualitative research that has been conducted related to rural surgery in the last decade. Although rural surgery is not a specialty unto itself, it has characteristics that set it apart from urban surgery, such as professional isolation,[1] being located long distances from additional health resources,[2] and differences in types and volumes of operative procedures.[3–8] Surgeons who practice in rural areas face different practice environments than do their urban counterparts, and this includes a different social context, one in which their patients are also frequently their friends and neighbors.[9,10] There are myriad facets of rural surgery to be explored, and different research questions require different research methods. Some are better suited to quantitative approaches, whereas others call for qualitative approaches.[11,12]

[a] Department of Population Health, University of Kansas School of Medicine, 3901 Rainbow Boulevard, MS 3044, Kansas City, KS 66160, USA; [b] Department of Surgery, University of Kansas School of Medicine, 3901 Rainbow Boulevard, MS 3044, Kansas City, KS 66160, USA
* Corresponding author. Department of Population Health, University of Kansas School of Medicine, 3901 Rainbow Boulevard, MS 3044, Kansas City, KS 66160.
E-mail address: dhughes5@kumc.edu

Surg Clin N Am 100 (2020) 949–970
https://doi.org/10.1016/j.suc.2020.05.011

Quantitative approaches to surgical research questions, through the use of surveys and analyses of large secondary databases, are far more commonly used,[13] which is understandable considering surgery's interests in patient outcomes, such as infection rates, length of stay, or mortality. Quantitative analysis techniques usually involve univariate statistics, common bivariate tests such as those that test for differences between groups, and regression models that take independent variables and work to predict an outcome of interest. However, quantitative data cannot capture the lived experiences of surgeons or patients.[11] Although quantitative methodologies can provide information about patterns occurring in large samples or at a population level, a qualitative approach can contextualize those patterns and begin to explain the nuances and reasons behind those patterns. Qualitative methodologies are the appropriate approach to answer many questions about structure, such as the circumstances in which an issue arises, and processes, the micro, meso, and macro level interactions of people over time in response to an issue.[12]

The intensive and demanding nature of surgery, along with the central task of cutting into other human beings, makes the study of the lived experiences of those involved critically important to all aspects of the profession, from training to operative skills and patient outcomes to surgeon wellness and beyond. In rural environments with tight-knit social fabrics, qualitative data related to surgical experiences are potentially even more meaningful. As surgeons and patients navigate their multiple, overlapping roles in their communities, they are simultaneously surgeons, patients, friends, neighbors, fellow professionals, town leaders, and more. Quantitative approaches are not well suited to studying such multi-layered social contexts. Therefore, the authors sought to assess how pervasive the use of qualitative methods has become, or not, across this potentially wide variety of topics.

METHODS

The authors searched the existing peer-reviewed literature using 3 database search engines: (1) MEDLINE, which also allowed inclusion of CINAHL Complete, Academic Search Premier, Business Source Premier, MasterFILE Premier, and PsycINFO; (2) PubMed; and (3) JSTOR. MEDLINE is a creation of the National Library of Medicine, and it covers subjects ranging from medicine and nursing to dentistry, veterinary medicine, and more. CINAHL Complete focuses on nursing and allied health subjects. Academic Search Premier is a broad, interdisciplinary source for scholarly references. Business Source Premier provides access to academic and industry publications focused, as the name suggests, on business. MasterFILE Premier was designed for public libraries and provides wide-ranging references, including periodicals, reference books, and primary source documents, as well as scholarly journals. PsycINFO is a product of the American Psychological Association and focuses on psychology and adjacent fields. PubMed is similar to MEDLINE but includes a wider range of sources on the life sciences and biomedical subjects. JSTOR is a database focusing on the social sciences, including sociology and the humanities.

The authors used these databases in order to include studies in major medical and surgical journals as well as journals oriented toward the social sciences that often publish health services research. The authors limited their results to articles published in English. Keywords used were "qualitative" AND "rural" AND "surgery." In the first 2 searches, advanced search options allowed the authors to narrow results to those with the keywords appearing in titles and/or abstracts. The MEDLINE search returned 131 results; when exact duplicates were automatically removed by the search engine, 67 remained. The PubMed search returned 72 results; PubMed does not automatically search for and remove exact duplicates. The JSTOR search was narrowed according to type of work and subject in order to restrict results to the biological sciences, general science, health policy, health sciences, population studies, or public health. Advanced search criteria in JSTOR do not permit isolating keywords in titles and/or abstracts; therefore, the authors applied their search terms to the full texts of articles. With these criteria in place, the JSTOR search initially yielded 138 results.

The initial MEDLINE, PubMed, and JSTOR searches together yielded 277 results, which were first examined for inclusion using titles, abstracts if available, and/or brief excerpts appearing in the search results. To meet the inclusion criteria, articles had to be original research studies whose subjects practiced or trained, received care, or lived in rural areas. The subjects had to be delivering or trained in surgical care or receiving or being asked about surgical care. These criteria ensured the included studies were of central importance to the field of rural surgery. To meet inclusion criteria specific to methodology, the articles had to demonstrate in the abstract and/or methods section that the authors collected and/or analyzed data using at least one of the following qualitative methods: participant observation, interviews, focus groups, or a combination. These criteria allowed for the inclusion of some mixed methods studies.

After manual removal of remaining duplicates within each search and this initial application of relevance and methodological criteria, 157 articles remained. The authors then compared the search results side by side in order to remove duplicates that appeared across the searches, which eliminated 54 articles, leaving 103. The authors analyzed these 103 articles in detail, using abstracts and full text to be certain they met the inclusion criteria outlined above. This more detailed review was necessary because, especially within the JSTOR results, abstracts were not always available, and brief excerpts in the search results did not always offer enough information to be certain about meeting inclusion criteria. In most cases, to determine whether an article met the methodological inclusion criteria, it was necessary to read the entire methods sections in the articles' full texts. Because the previous issue of this journal focusing on rural surgery was published in 2009, the authors viewed this as an update on research that has been conducted since that time and therefore limited their results to the years 2010 to 2019. This limitation excluded 8 articles. The authors' final results consisted of 46 original research articles that were qualitative or mixed methods, were conducted in the previous decade, and were meaningfully relevant to rural surgery in the United States and across the globe. The authors have detailed their search process and the application of their review criteria in **Table 1**.

RESULTS

The authors' review included 46 articles spanning the years 2010 to 2019, as of December 2019 (Appendix 1). Nearly half the articles in the final sample included subjects who were people living in rural areas being asked about surgical conditions or services (n = 22, 47.8%), and the other half studied subjects who were rural health care practitioners of various training levels and specialties (n = 23, 50.0%). One study was included because its subjects practiced in urban areas but provided care to those who lived in rural areas (n = 1, 2.2%). The authors categorized these 46 articles by content in 2 different ways: by surgical area involved in the study and by primary topic explored.

Surgical Areas Investigated

In terms of surgical area investigated by the studies, around one-third (n = 14, 30.4%) of the articles did not specify a particular subspecialty area. The next most-frequently

Table 1
Search criteria and results

	Search 1: Medline	Search 2: PubMed	Search 3: JSTOR	Total
Search criteria	"qualitative" AND "rural" AND "surgery" in title/abstract; 2010–2019	"qualitative" AND "rural" AND "surgery" in abstract; 2010–2019	"qualitative" AND " rural" AND "surgery" in full text; 2010–2019	
Additional criteria	No	No	Subjects limited to: biological sciences, general science, health policy, health sciences, population studies, and public health	
Initial results	131	72	138	341
Duplicates automatically removed by search engine	67	72	138	277
Manual removal of duplicates within each search and initial application of criteria for relevance and methodology	50	56	41	157
Removal of duplicates across searches	(44 in both Medline and PubMed) 6 only in Medline	12 only in PubMed	No overlap with other searches	
	62		41	103
Final results after detailed application of criteria for relevance and methodology using abstracts and full text				46

studied surgical area was obstetrics and gynecology (n = 9, 19.6%). The authors included studies regarding genital surgery in the obstetrics category, because they pertained to women's health as well. The third most-frequent surgical area was surgical oncology (n = 5, 10.9%). Surgical areas are cross-tabulated with primary topics in **Table 2.**

Of the studies covering unspecified types of surgery, 12 of 14 focused on the provision of surgical care in rural areas and included the logistics of providing care in rural areas, perceptions of access, and community input on types of services needed. The other 2 studies in this category discussed surgical training and operating room (OR) safety.

Within obstetrics and gynecology, 3 of 9 studies explored postoperative lived experiences; 3 studies explored how patients made or would make care decisions, and 3

Table 2
Cross-tabulation of surgical areas and topics covered by articles included in this review

	Topic										
Surgical Area	Providing Surgical Service in Rural Areas	Patient Decision Making	Postoperative Experiences	Surgical Skills	Disease Experience	Practice Location Choice	Program Evaluation	Ethics	OR Safety	Surgical Training	Total (%)
Surgery, unspecified	12	0	0	0	0	0	0	0	1	1	14 (30.4)
Obstetric and genital surgery	1	3	3	1	1	0	0	0	0	0	9 (19.6)
Surgical oncology	1	3	1	0	0	0	0	0	0	0	5 (10.9)
General surgery	0	0	1	2	0	1	0	0	0	0	4 (8.7)
Ophthalmologic surgery	0	3	0	0	1	0	0	0	0	0	4 (8.7)
General practitioner surgery	2	0	0	0	0	0	0	0	0	0	2 (4.4)
Orthopedic surgery	0	0	1	0	0	0	1	0	0	0	2 (4.4)
Transplant surgery	1	0	1	0	0	0	0	0	0	0	2 (4.4)
Cardiac surgery	0	0	0	0	0	0	1	1	0	0	2 (4.4)
Colorectal surgery	0	1	0	0	0	0	0	0	0	0	1 (2.2)
Not clinical	0	0	0	0	0	1	0	0	0	0	1 (2.2)
Total	17 (37.0%)	10 (21.7%)	7 (15.2%)	3 (6.5%)	2 (4.4%)	2 (4.4%)	2 (4.4%)	1 (2.2%)	1 (2.2%)	1 (2.2%)	46

studies explored each of the following: lived experiences of disease, surgical skills needed, and the provision of surgical care in rural areas.

Within surgical oncology, most studies (3 of 5) focused on how patients made or would make care decisions. One article explored postoperative lived experiences, and 1 article explored the provision of care in rural areas.

Research Subjects

There were 15 studies (32.6%) that collected data from patients only. An additional 6 studies included patients as well as other groups, for a total of 21 studies (45.7%) that included at least some patients. There were 7 studies (15.2%) that used surgeons only. An additional 6 studies included surgeons as well as others, for a total of 13 studies (28.3%) that included at least some surgeons.

Variation in Data Collection

Regarding data collection methods, over half of the studies exclusively used interviews (n = 25, 54.4%). Five studies exclusively used focus groups (10.9%). Six studies used a combination of qualitative methods (13.0%), and 10 were mixed methods studies (21.7%). The authors defined "mixed methods" as any study that used at least 1 quantitative method and at least 1 qualitative method, together, in data collection, data analysis, or both. The authors based their categorization of data collection methods on wording used by each study's authors. The words "interviews," "focus groups," and "mixed methods" were used consistently, but wording used to describe observation, participant observation, and qualitative surveys was less consistent. The latter 3 methods were never used alone, only in conjunction with another qualitative or quantitative methods. **Table 3** shows a cross-tabulation of data collection and data analysis methods used in these 46 studies.

Variation in Data Analysis

Several paradigms and approaches to qualitative analysis were used in the articles included in the authors' sample. The most common approach to data analysis was thematic analysis (n = 18, 39.1%). This is an approach to qualitative analysis that identifies and reports patterns in the data.[14] The next most common approach explicitly stated in the authors' articles was grounded theory (n = 9, 19.6%), an

Table 3
Cross-tabulation of studies' data collection and analysis methods

	Data Analysis Methods					
Data Collection Methods	**Thematic Analysis**	**Other Inductive Methods**	**Grounded Theory**	**Deductive Methods**	**Unspecified**	**Total (%)**
Interviews only	8	8	4	3	2	25 (54.4)
Focus groups only	3	0	2	0	0	5 (10.9)
Multiple qualitative methods	3	2	1	0	0	6 (13.0)
Mixed methods (quantitative and qualitative)	4	1	2	1	2	10 (21.7)
Total	18 (39.1%)	11 (23.9%)	9 (19.6%)	4 (8.7%)	4 (8.7%)	46 (100.0)

approach stemming from the field of sociology that aims to build theoretical explanations of processes that are grounded closely in the data.[15,16] There were 11 articles (23.9%) that used other inductive approaches: connecting and categorizing (n = 1); the constant comparative method (n = 1), which overlaps with grounded theory content analysis[17] (n = 1), a method to code and categorize text;[18] the Delphi method (n = 1), a technique that invites expert opinion through a series of questionnaires;[19] and phenomenology (n = 2), an analytical approach with its roots in European philosophy used when interested in sense-making around the lived experience of a certain phenomenon.[16] A few studies used deductive methods of analysis, such as an a priori codebook (n = 4). The authors used the articles' own descriptions of their analytical techniques to categorize the studies. When descriptions did not fit a known qualitative approach, usually because of vague wording, studies were deemed to have used "unspecified" data analysis methods (n = 4).

Most of the studies (n = 37, 80.4%) did not appear in surgical journals. Six (13.0%) appeared in journals dedicated to rural issues. Nearly one-third of studies collected data from research subjects in Africa (n = 15, 32.6%). Australians and North Americans were the subjects of 12 studies each (26.1% each). In North America, the United States and Canada were represented equally, with 6 studies each. **Table 4** lists all countries and continents represented by studies meeting the authors' inclusion criteria.

DISCUSSION

To address questions pertinent to rural surgery, qualitative researchers have primarily used interviews, engaged patients as subjects of this research, and used thematic

Table 4
Countries represented by studies included in this review

Country (or Countries)	N (%)	Continent	N (%)
Australia and New Zealand	1 (2.2%)	Australia	12 (26.1)
Australia	11 (23.9%)		
Ethiopia	1 (2.2%)	Africa	15 (32.6)
Ghana	2 (4.4%)		
Kenya	1 (2.2%)		
Malawi	2 (4.4%)		
Niger	1 (2.2%)		
Nigeria	1 (2.2%)		
Rwanda	1 (2.2%)		
Sierra Leone	1 (2.2%)		
South Africa	2 (4.4%)		
Uganda	2 (4.4%)		
Zambia	1 (2.2%)		
Bangladesh	1 (2.2%)	Asia	2 (4.4)
China	1 (2.2%)		
Sweden	2 (4.4%)	Europe	3 (6.5)
United Kingdom	1 (2.2%)		
Canada	6 (13.0%)	North America	12 (26.1)
United States	6 (13.0%)		
Low- or middle-income countries	2 (4.4%)	Multiple	2 (4.4)
Total	46 (100.0%)	Total	46 (100.0)

analysis methods. Surgical journals are not currently the primary venues for these types of studies; instead, they were published in a variety of specialty-specific or geography-specific journals.

Qualitative methods are best suited for answering research questions about why and how.[11,12] These methods allow for a deeper understanding of context, which is particularly helpful to the goal of improving the delivery of surgical services.[20] Surgery is resource intensive, so it follows that more than one-third of studies investigated the provision of surgery broadly in rural areas. Surgery is physical and intimate in ways some other specialties are not, making a shared understanding of social context crucial for surgeons, patients, and communities alike. This reality is reflected in the large proportion of studies focusing on how patients make care decisions and what their postoperative or disease-related lived experiences have been.

Because this review focuses on the application of qualitative research specifically to rural surgery, it is fairly narrow in scope. Many qualitative studies about surgery and surgical education exist and have been published but did not meet the authors' inclusion criteria. A recent article by Maragh-Bass and colleagues,[20] the first review to systematically detail the use of qualitative research in surgery, included 878 articles. Similar to the authors' findings, their review found that interviews were the most common method of data collection. Unlike the authors' findings, the review of Maragh-Bass and colleagues found the most frequently used qualitative approaches for data analysis were grounded theory and phenomenology. Their review also showed a high frequency of content analysis but did not include a category for thematic analysis, whereas the authors' review showed frequent usage of thematic analysis. This discrepancy demonstrates a need for clear definitions of qualitative methodologies to be applied uniformly across health services research so that the results of studies that use the same analytical processes may be better compared.

There are several reasons for the large difference in number of studies in the Maragh-Bass and colleagues review (n = 878) and the authors' review (n = 46). The authors' review was limited to 2010 to present, whereas the previous review included articles published from 1983 to 2015. The authors also focused exclusively on rural surgery, as stated. It is interesting, though, that the application of the authors' "relevance to rural" criteria appears to be what so greatly reduced the authors' number of results.

The low incidence of qualitative rural surgery research may be related to the nature of qualitative research itself. Corbin and Strauss[12] outline several reasons researchers pursue qualitative methods rather than quantitative methods:

> ... *[T]o explore the inner experiences of participants," "to explore how meanings are formed and transformed," "to explore areas not yet thoroughly researched," "to discover relevant variables that later can be tested through quantitative research," and "to take a holistic and comprehensive approach to the study of a phenomena.*[12]

The authors' results show the first reason, exploration of "inner experiences," is occurring in rural surgery research, as investigators strive to understand patients' experiences through interviews and focus groups. However, they saw less evidence of studies addressing meanings in the context of rural surgery. The large proportion of studies based in low- and middle-income countries could represent rural surgery researchers seeking new areas of research and working to discover variables needing further testing. However, it could also be reflective of discussions in the profession that rural surgery is global surgery. There is a sense that the two may be synonymous in terms of their resource needs and logistical challenges.[21]

The low incidence of qualitative rural surgery studies may also be attributable to existing publication trends. Medical and surgical publications typically focus on quantitative studies, and their audiences are more accustomed to evaluating the quality of quantitative methods. A review by Gagliardi and Dobrow[13] showed that in the years 1999 to 2008, major general medical journals ranged from 0.0% to 6.4% in their frequency of qualitative study publication. In that light, it is not surprising that when the scope of a review is narrowed not only to surgery, but also to rural surgery, the results are scarce.

Further Research: Surgical Areas

Given the current surgical workforce shortage,[22] which is particularly acute in rural areas,[23,24] there may also be a need to further explore the makeup of surgical teams. This review suggests that outside the United States, there are general practitioners or other nonsurgeons performing surgical procedures. Regardless of country, qualitative approaches could be used to better understand how practitioners of varying education and training levels can work together across the perioperative services continuum to best serve rural patients.[25,26] In addition, qualitative research into practice location decisions of surgical trainees and practicing surgeons, as well as the lived experiences of surgeons and their family members in rural areas, will continue to be important as the surgical profession works to address the rural surgeon shortage.

The authors' results suggest that understudied areas relevant to rural surgery may be surgeons' and other surgical care providers' experiences working in teams, skills needed for rural surgery, surgical training experiences (such as general surgery residency), and ethical issues, such as surgery in the context of end-of-life care. Only a few of the studies in the authors' review examined these or similar areas, such as OR safety,[27] surgical skills and training,[28–31] and the ethics of medical volunteerism.[32] These areas need investigation especially considering that rural populations tend to be older and sicker, and the health care needs of the baby boomer generation continue to build. In that context, cardiac surgery stands out among the authors' results as a nascent area in current rural surgery research,[32,33] and it merits further qualitative investigation. Similar to obstetrics, potential areas of qualitative investigation could center on patient experiences of access or barriers to timely care and the role of family members in care decisions.

In terms of surgical specialties, obstetrics, including genital surgery, appeared most frequently in these results. Considering childbirth and rituals around women's health are not only intensely personal, but also deeply connected to constructs such as family, tradition, and cultural values,[34–38] it is an area well-suited for qualitative inquiry. The authors' review suggests qualitative researchers are actively pursuing research questions in rural obstetrics, such as how obstetric emergencies are identified and handled,[36,39] women's experiences with obstetric fistula,[34,35,40] the role of male partners in obstetric decisions,[38] and how to improve patient experiences of gynecologic cancer treatment.[41] Obstetrics procedures are often time sensitive, a characteristic even more salient in rural areas, where distance from additional health resources may produce an insurmountable barrier to timely care. This review suggests that most qualitative work related to obstetric patients' experiences, the roles of their family members in obstetrics decision, and how barriers to care are experienced, is taking place outside of the United States, but there is a need for exploration of these topics within the United States as well.

Another surgical topic related to the aging population that does not appear in the authors' results is patient experiences with surgery in the context of multiple comorbidities. Although the authors' results included several instances of lived experiences with a single disease, or the lived experience of a single surgical operation, it is increasingly likely that patients, including those in rural areas, will experience surgical care in the context of multiple health conditions.

Several structural barriers exist for rural surgery research. For example, most research comes from academic institutions, many of which are in urban areas. Research requires time and money; travel time from urban institutions to rural areas may or may not be possible, and money may or may not be available for travel expenses and other qualitative research costs, such as transcription. Qualitative research itself also faces barriers: medical schools have only 4 years to educate students on how to be doctors. They have limited time for research methods in their curricula, and given the aforementioned trends in publication and funding, the odds are that schools would choose to focus on quantitative methods. According to the Association for American Medical Colleges, in academic year 2016 to 2017, there were 145 medical schools that responded to a survey about their student research requirements. Sixty-two schools (42.8%) had a research requirement. The survey asked which categories of research would satisfy students' research requirements; the categories were basic science (biomedical), biology/chemistry/physics, bioengineering/informatics, clinical, translational, public health/health services, and ethics/humanities/social sciences. Of the 62 responding schools, 60 (96.8%) allowed students to do public health/health services research, and 50 (80.6%) allowed ethics/humanities/social sciences research, 2 fields that could be more likely to use qualitative methods.[42] However, knowing projects are allowed in these areas does not help us understand what training students are given in relevant research methodologies.

For qualitative research of rural surgical topics to occur, either surgeons need to find research partners who are qualitative experts or there need to be qualitative experts who are interested in pursuing surgery-oriented research questions. In the first scenario, surgeons needing qualitatively trained partners, academic and community surgeons alike may or may not have the resources to compensate these partners. In the United States, there is increasing pressure for researchers to earn extramural funding, and over time, competition for National Institutes of Health dollars in particular has grown increasingly fierce.[43] In the second scenario, for qualitative experts to be interested in surgical questions, there need to be institutions that hire qualitative experts and give them access to surgeons and surgery. The natural environment would be academic medical centers, but this results in circular logic that leads us back to urban locations and funding pressures. Given these structural issues, the dearth of rural surgical research in the United States is not surprising.

Academic institutions not only produce research but also are responsible for the education and training of surgeons. The lack of surgical education research that is related to rural surgery is again likely due to structure: most medical schools and surgery residencies are in urban locations. If researchers want to study surgeons or surgical trainees, they are almost always doing so in urban areas. There are, of course, medical schools and surgery residency programs that are located on regional campuses, offer rural rotations to third- and fourth-year medical students, and feature rural tracks in their training programs. However, these rural offerings are the exception, not the rule.[44,45]

The evidence in this review shows that topics pertinent to rural surgery, such as teamwork, rural surgical skills, training experiences, and ethical issues, merit further investigation, and they are all areas well-suited for exploration using qualitative methods. If future qualitative work on these topics is to be useful to rural surgery as a profession, conceptually and in practice, it must be rigorous. The studies included in this review varied widely in their methodological rigor. In some cases, rigor could not be assessed because the investigators were insufficiently transparent. Four studies (8.7%) did not specify their data analysis methods in enough detail for their approach to be categorized.[28,33,46,47] Without this specificity, the authors could not speak to their findings' credibility, transferability, or integrity of the research process.[48] Many journals provide guidelines for submitting qualitative research, and the increasing use of reporting checklists, like the Consolidated Criteria for Reporting Qualitative Research (COREQ)[49] or the Standards for Reporting Qualitative Research (SRQR),[50] may help improve the quality of qualitative work as well as the trust and confidence in qualitative work more generally.

The authors' inclusion and exclusion criteria limited their sample of reviewed articles to 46. The authors only included articles published in English and articles published in 2010 or later. Part of the contribution of this article is an assessment of the prevalence of qualitative work related to rural surgery, but the authors acknowledge that much qualitative research has been conducted in adjacent content areas but was not included in this review. In addition, some categorizations concerning methods were challenging given the lack of information that investigators provided, but the authors have detailed the reasoning behind their categorization above.

The authors' systematic search of peer-reviewed, published work pertaining to rural surgery using qualitative methods yielded 46 articles that fit their inclusion criteria. The authors have described the surgical areas, methodological approaches, types of subjects, and geographic locations of the studies. The authors also discussed barriers to both rural surgery research and qualitative research, which taken together help to explain the sparse number of articles fitting their inclusion criteria. Future rural surgery research efforts should consider using qualitative methods because of their unique ability to address key questions, such as surgical teamwork, workforce issues, and the aging of the rural patient population.

DISCLOSURE

The authors have nothing to disclose.

REFERENCES

1. Heneghan SJ, Bordley J, Dietz PA, et al. Comparison of urban and rural general surgeons: motivations for practice location, practice patterns, and education requirements. J Am Coll Surg 2005;201(5):732–6.
2. Ahmed N, Conn LG, Chiu M, et al. Career satisfaction among general surgeons in Canada: a qualitative study of enablers and barriers to improve recruitment and retention in general surgery. Acad Med 2012;87(11):1616–21.
3. Finlayson SRG. Surgery in rural America. Surg Innov 2005;12(4):299–305.
4. Valentine RJ, Jones A, Biester TW, et al. General surgery workloads and practice patterns in the United States, 2007 to 2009: a 10-year update from the American Board of Surgery. Ann Surg 2011;254(3):520–6.
5. Cogbill TH, Cofer JB, Jarman BT. Contemporary issues in rural surgery. Curr Probl Surg 2012;49(5):263–318.
6. Stiles R, Reyes J, Helmer SD, et al. What procedures are rural general surgeons performing and are they prepared to perform specialty procedures in practice? Am Surg 2019;85(6):587–94.
7. Deal SB, Cook MR, Hughes D, et al. Training for a career in rural and nonmetropolitan surgery-a practical needs assessment. J Surg Educ 2018;75(6):e229–33.

8. Doescher MP, Jackson JE, Fordyce MA, et al. Variability in general surgical procedures in rural and urban U.S. hospital inpatient settings. Seattle (WA): WWAMI Rural Health Research Center; 2015. p. 1–12. Final Report #142.
9. Kilpatrick S, Cheers B, Gilles M, et al. Boundary crossers, communities, and health: exploring the role of rural health professionals. Health Place 2008; 15(2009):284–90.
10. Brooks K, Eley D, Pratt R, et al. Management of professional boundaries in rural practice. Acad Med 2012;87(8):1091–5.
11. Pope C, Mays N. Reaching the parts other methods cannot reach: an introduction to qualitative methods in health and health services research. BMJ 1995; 311:42–5.
12. Corbin J, Strauss A. Basics of qualitative research: techniques and procedures for developing grounded theory. 4th edition. Thousand Oaks (CA): SAGE Publications Ltd; 2015.
13. Gagliardi AR, Dobrow MJ. Paucity of qualitative research in general medical and health services and policy research journals: analysis of publication rates. BMC Health Serv Res 2011;11(268):1–7.
14. Braun V, Clarke V. Using thematic analysis in psychology. Qual Res Psychol 2006; 3(2):77–101.
15. Glaser B, Strauss A. The discovery of grounded theory: strategies for qualitative research. New Brunswick (Canada): Aldine Transaction; 1999.
16. Starks H, Trinidad SB. Choose your method: a comparison of phenomenology, discourse analysis, and grounded theory. Qual Health Res 2007;17(10):1372–80.
17. Glaser BG. The constant comparative method of qualitative analysis. Social Probl 1965;12(4):436–45.
18. Vaismoradi M, Turunen H, Bondas T. Content analysis and thematic analysis: implications for conducting a qualitative descriptive study. Nurs Health Sci 2013; 15(3):398–405.
19. Delphi method. 2020. Available at: https://www.rand.org/topics/delphi-method.html. Accessed January 30, 2020.
20. Maragh-Bass AC, Appelson JR, Changoor NR, et al. Prioritizing qualitative research in surgery: a synthesis and analysis of publication trends. Surgery 2016;160(6):1447–55.
21. Meara JG, Leather AJ, Hagander L, et al. Global surgery 2030: evidence and solutions for achieving health, welfare, and economic development. Lancet 2015; 386:569–624.
22. Ellison EC, Pawlik TM, Way DP, et al. Ten-year reassessment of the shortage of general surgeons: increases in graduation numbers of general surgery residents are insufficient to meet the future demand for general surgeons. Surgery 2018; 164:726–32.
23. Lynge DC, Larson EH. Workforce issues in rural surgery. Surg Clin North Am 2009;89(2009):1285–91.
24. Christian Lynge D, Larson EH, Thompson MJ, et al. A longitudinal analysis of the general surgery workforce in the united states, 1981-2005. Arch Surg 2008; 143(4):345–50.
25. Swayne A, Eley DS. Synergy and sustainability in rural procedural medicine: views from the coalface. Aust J Rural Health 2010;18(1):38–42.
26. Abbot B, Laurence C, Elliott T. GP surgeons: what are they? An audit of GP surgeons in South Australia. Rural Remote Health 2014;14(3):2585.

27. Sandelin A, Gustafsson BÅ, Kalman S. Prerequisites for safe intraoperative nursing care and teamwork—Operating theatre nurses' perspectives: a qualitative interview study. J Clin Nurs 2019;28(13/14):2635–43.
28. Goudie C, Shanahan J, Gill A, et al. Investigating the efficacy of anatomical silicone models developed from a 3D printed mold for perineal repair suturing simulation. Cureus 2018;10(8):e3181.
29. Hoops HE, Deveney KE, Brasel KJ. Development of an assessment tool for surgeons in their first year of independent practice: the junior surgeon performance assessment tool. J Surg Educ 2019;76(6):e199–208.
30. Hoops HE, Burt MR, Deveney K, et al. What they may not tell you and you may not know to ask: what is expected of surgeons in their first year of independent practice. J Surg Educ 2018;75(6):e134–41.
31. Liang R, Dornan T, Nestel D. Why do women leave surgical training? A qualitative and feminist study. Lancet 2019;393(10171):541–9.
32. Coors ME, Matthew TL, Matthew DB. Ethical precepts for medical volunteerism: including local voices and values to guide RHD surgery in Rwanda. J Med Ethics 2015;41(10):814–9.
33. Courtney-Pratt H, Johnson C, Cameron-Tucker H, et al. Investigating the feasibility of promoting and sustaining delivery of cardiac rehabilitation in a rural community. Rural Remote Health 2012;12:1838.
34. Kaplan JA, Kandodo J, Sclafani J, et al. An investigation of the relationship between autonomy, childbirth practices, and obstetric fistula among women in rural Lilongwe District, Malawi. BMC Int Health Hum Rights 2017;17:1–10.
35. Bashah DT, Worku AG, Yitayal M, et al. The loss of dignity: social experience and coping of women with obstetric fistula, in Northwest Ethiopia. BMC Womens Health 2019;19(1):84.
36. Khan R, Blum LS, Sultana M, et al. An examination of women experiencing obstetric complications requiring emergency care: perceptions and sociocultural consequences of caesarean sections in Bangladesh. J Health Popul Nutr 2012;30(2): 159–71.
37. Scorgie F, Beksinska M, Chersich M, et al. "Cutting for love": genital incisions to enhance sexual desirability and commitment in KwaZulu-Natal, South Africa. Reprod Health Matters 2010;18(35):64–73.
38. Story WT, Barrington C, Fordham C, et al. Male involvement and accommodation during obstetric emergencies in rural Ghana: a qualitative analysis. Int Perspect Sex Reprod Health 2016;42(4):211–9.
39. Oiyemhonlan B, Udofia E, Punguyire D. Identifying obstetrical emergencies at Kintampo Municipal Hospital: a perspective from pregnant women and nursing midwives. Afr J Reprod Health 2013;17(2):129–40.
40. Khisa AM, Nyamongo IK. Still living with fistula: an exploratory study of the experience of women with obstetric fistula following corrective surgery in West Pokot, Kenya. Reprod Health Matters 2012;20(40):59–66.
41. Wainer J, Willis E, Dwyer J, et al. The treatment experiences of Australian women with gynaecological cancers and how they can be improved: a qualitative study. Reprod Health Matters 2012;20(40):38–48.
42. Medical student research requirement: types of research. 2018. Available at: https://www.aamc.org/data-reports/curriculum-reports/interactive-data/medical-student-research-requirement-us-medical-schools. Accessed January 29, 2020.
43. Dolgin E. The young and the restless. Nature 2017;551(7678):S15–8.

44. Rossi IR, Wiegmann AL, Schou P, et al. Reap what you sow: which rural surgery training programs currently exist and do medical students know of their existence. J Surg Educ 2018;75(3):697–701.
45. Rural Surgery Program. Section III: surgical specialties [Website]. 2018. Available at: https://www.facs.org/education/resources/residency-search/specialties/rural. Accessed September 2, 2018.
46. Gwala-Ngozo J, Taylor M, Aldous C. Understanding the experiences of doctors who undertake elective surgery on HIV/AIDS patients in an area of high incidence in South Africa. Afr J AIDS Res 2010;9(1):11–6.
47. Raykar NP, Yorlets RR, Liu C, et al. A qualitative study exploring contextual challenges to surgical care provision in 21 LMICs. Lancet 2015;385(Suppl 2):S15.
48. Devers KJ. How will we know "good" qualitative research when we see it? Beginning the dialogue in health services research. Health Serv Res 1999;34(5): 1153–86.
49. Tong A, Sainsbury P, Craig J. Consolidated criteria for reporting qualitative research (COREQ): a 32-item checklist for interviews and focus groups. Int J Qual Health Care 2007;19(6):349–57.
50. O'Brien BC, Harris IB, Beckman TJ, et al. Standards for reporting qualitative research: a synthesis of recommendations. Acad Med 2014;89(9): 1245–51.
51. Alami H, Fortin J-P, Gagnon M-P, et al. The challenges of a complex and innovative telehealth project: a qualitative evaluation of the Eastern Quebec Telepathology Network. Int J Health Policy Manag 2018;7(5):421–32.
52. Cook MR, Hughes D, Deal SB, et al. When rural is no longer rural: demand for subspecialty trained surgeons increases with increasing population of a non-metropolitan area. Am J Surg 2019;218(5):1022–7.
53. Eley DS, Synnott R, Baker PG, et al. A decade of Australian Rural Clinical School graduates–where are they and why? Rural Remote Health 2012;12:1937.
54. Gajewski J, Mweemba C, Cheelo M, et al. Non-physician clinicians in rural Africa: lessons from the Medical Licentiate programme in Zambia. Hum Resour Health 2017;15:1–9.
55. Gajewski J, Bijlmakers L, Mwapasa G, et al. 'I think we are going to leave these cases'. Obstacles to surgery in rural Malawi: a qualitative study of provider perspectives. Trop Med Int Health 2018;23(10):1141–7.
56. Groen RS, Sriram VM, Kamara TB, et al. Individual and community perceptions of surgical care in Sierra Leone. Trop Med Int Health 2014;19(1):107–16.
57. Hughes D, Cook MR, Deal SB, et al. Rural surgeons' perspectives on necessity of post-residency training are stable across generations. Am J Surg 2019;217(2): 296–300.
58. Humber N, Dickinson P. Rural patients' experiences accessing surgery in British Columbia. Can J Surg 2010;53(6):373–8.
59. Lindseth GN, Denny DL. Patients' experiences with cholecystitis and a cholecystectomy. Gastroenterol Nurs 2014;37(6):407–14.
60. McGrath P, Holewa H. 'It's a regional thing': financial impact of renal transplantation on live donors. Rural Remote Health 2012;12:2144.
61. Nostedt MC, McKay AM, Hochman DJ, et al. The location of surgical care for rural patients with rectal cancer: patterns of treatment and patient perspectives. Can J Surg 2014;57(6):398–404.
62. Nwanna-Nzewunwa OC, Ajiko M-M, Kirya F, et al. Barriers and facilitators of surgical care in rural Uganda: a mixed methods study. J Surg Res 2016;204:242–50.

63. Palmer SL, Winskell K, Patterson AE, et al. 'A living death': a qualitative assessment of quality of life among women with trichiasis in rural Niger. Int Health 2014; 6:291–7.
64. Parker V, Bellamy D, Rossiter R, et al. The experiences of head and neck cancer patients requiring major surgery. Cancer Nurs 2014;37(4):263–70.
65. Phillips JJ, Beyeza T, Okello J, et al. Orthopaedic outreach program in Uganda: a strategy to improve inequality in service delivery between rural and urban communities. East Cent Afr J Surg 2010;15(2):3–9.
66. Poland F, Spalding N, Gregory S, et al. Developing patient education to enhance recovery after colorectal surgery through action research: a qualitative study. BMJ Open 2017;7(6):e013498.
67. Raykar NP, Yorlets RR, Liu C, et al. The how project: understanding contextual challenges to global surgical care provision in low-resource settings. BMJ Glob Health 2016;1(4):e000075.
68. Ristevski E, Regan M, Birks D, et al. A qualitative study of rural women's views for the treatment of early breast cancer. Health Expect 2015;18(6):2928–40.
69. Segevall C, Söderberg S, Björkman Randström K. The journey toward taking the day for granted again: the experiences of rural older people's recovery from hip fracture surgery. Orthop Nurs 2019;38(6):359–66.
70. Smith Z, Leslie G, Wynaden D. Australian perioperative nurses' experiences of assisting in multi-organ procurement surgery: a grounded theory study. Int J Nurs Stud 2015;52(3):705–15.
71. Tafida A, Gilbert C. Exploration of indigenous knowledge systems in relation to couching in Nigeria. Afr Vis Eye Health 2016;75(1):1–6.
72. Wade VA, Eliott JA, Hiller JE. A qualitative study of ethical, medico-legal and clinical governance matters in Australian telehealth services. J Telemed Telecare 2012;18(2):109–14.
73. Wright FC, Gagliardi AR, Fraser N, et al. Adoption of surgical innovations: factors influencing use of sentinel lymph node biopsy for breast cancer. Surg Innov 2011; 18(4):379–86.
74. Youl P, Morris B, Jenny A, et al. What factors influence the treatment decisions of women with breast cancer? Does residential location play a role? Rural Remote Health 2019;19(2):4497.
75. Zhang M, Wu X, Li L, et al. Understanding barriers to cataract surgery among older persons in rural China through focus groups. Ophthalmic Epidemiol 2011;18(4):179–86.

APPENDIX 1: ARTICLES INCLUDED IN SYSTEMATIC REVIEW

First Author, y	Title	Journal	Country Represented
Abbot et al,[26] 2014	GP surgeons: what are they? An audit of GP surgeons in South Australia	*Rural and Remote Health*	Australia

(continued)

First Author, y	Title	Journal	Country Represented
Ahmed et al,[2] 2012	Career satisfaction among general surgeons in Canada: a qualitative study of enablers and barriers to improve recruitment and retention in general surgery	*Academic Medicine*	Canada
Alami et al,[51] 2018	The challenges of a complex and innovative telehealth project: a qualitative evaluation of the Eastern Quebec Telepathology Network	*International Journal of Health Policy and Management*	Canada
Bashah et al,[35] 2019	The loss of dignity: social experience and coping of women with obstetric fistula, in northwest Ethiopia	*BMC Women's Health*	Ethiopia
Cook et al,[52] 2019	When rural is no longer rural: demand for subspecialty trained surgeons increases with increasing population of a nonmetropolitan area	*American Journal of Surgery*	US
Coors et al,[32] 2015	Ethical precepts for medical volunteerism: including local voices and values to guide RHD surgery in Rwanda	*Journal of Medical Ethics*	Rwanda
Courtney-Pratt et al,[33] 2012	Investigating the feasibility of promoting and sustaining delivery of cardiac rehabilitation in a rural community	*Rural and Remote Health*	Australia
Deal et al,[7] 2018	Training for a career in rural and	*Journal of Surgical Education*	US

(continued)

First Author, y	Title	Journal	Country Represented
	nonmetropolitan surgery—a practical needs assessment		
Eley et al,[53] 2012	A decade of Australian Rural Clinical School graduates—where are they and why?	*Rural and Remote Health*	Australia
Gajewski et al,[54] 2017	Non-physician clinicians in rural Africa: lessons from the Medical Licentiate programme in Zambia	*Human Resources for Health*	Zambia
Gajewski et al,[55] 2018	"I think we are going to leave these cases." Obstacles to surgery in rural Malawi: a qualitative study of provider perspectives	*Tropical Medicine and International Health*	Malawi
Goudie et al,[28] 2018	Investigating the efficacy of anatomical silicone models developed from a 3D printed mold for perineal repair suturing simulation	*Cureus*	Canada
Groen et al,[56] 2014	Individual and community perceptions of surgical care in Sierra Leone	*Tropical Medicine and International Health*	Sierra Leone
Gwala-Ngozo et al,[46] 2010	Understanding the experiences of doctors who undertake elective surgery on HIV/AIDS patients in an area of high incidence in South Africa	*African Journal of AIDS Research*	South Africa
Hoops et al,[30] 2018	Development of an assessment tool for surgeons in	*Journal of Surgical Education*	US

(continued)

First Author, y	Title	Journal	Country Represented
	their first year of independent practice		
Hoops et al,[29] 2019	What they may not tell you and you may not know to ask: what is expected of surgeons in their first year of independent practice	*Journal of Surgical Education*	US
Hughes et al,[57] 2019	Rural surgeons' perspectives on necessity of post-residency training are stable across generations	*American Journal of Surgery*	US
Humber & Dickinson,[58] 2010	Rural patients' experiences accessing surgery in British Columbia	*Canadian Journal of Surgery*	Canada
Kaplan et al,[34] 2017	An investigation of the relationship between autonomy, childbirth practices, and obstetric fistula among women in rural Lilongwe District, Malawi	*BMC International Health and Human Rights*	Malawi
Khan et al,[36] 2012	An examination of women experiencing obstetric complications requiring emergency care: perceptions and sociocultural consequences of caesarean sections in Bangladesh	*Journal of Health, Population and Nutrition*	Bangladesh
Khisa & Nyamongo,[40] 2012	Still living with fistula: an exploratory study of the experience of women with	*Reproductive Health Matters*	Kenya

(continued)

First Author, y	Title	Journal	Country Represented
	obstetric fistula following corrective surgery in West Pokot, Kenya		
Liang et al,[31] 2019	Why do women leave surgical training? A qualitative and feminist study	*Lancet*	Australia and New Zealand
Lindseth & Denny,[59] 2014	Patients' experiences with cholecystitis and a cholecystectomy	*Gastroenterology Nursing*	US
McGrath & Holewa,[60] 2012	"It's a regional thing": financial impact of renal transplantation on live donors	*Rural and Remote Health*	Australia
Nostedt et al,[61] 2014	The location of surgical care for rural patients with rectal cancer: patterns of treatment and patient perspectives	*Canadian Journal of Surgery*	Canada
Nwanna-Nzewunwa et al,[62] 2016	Barriers and facilitators of surgical care in rural Uganda: a mixed methods study	*Journal of Surgical Research*	Uganda
Oiyemhonlan et al,[39] 2013	Identifying obstetrical emergencies at Kintampo Municipal Hospital: a perspective from pregnant women and nursing midwives	*African Journal of Reproductive Health*	Ghana
Palmer et al,[63] 2014	"A living death": a qualitative assessment of quality of life among women with trichiasis in rural Niger	*International Health*	Niger

(continued)

First Author, y	Title	Journal	Country Represented
Parker et al,[64] 2014	The experiences of head and neck cancer patients requiring major surgery	*Cancer Nursing*	Australia
Phillips et al,[65] 2010	Orthopaedic outreach program in Uganda: a strategy to improve inequality in service delivery between rural and urban communities	*East and Central African Journal of Surgery*	Uganda
Poland et al,[66] 2017	Developing patient education to enhance recovery after colorectal surgery through action research: a qualitative study	*BMJ Open*	UK
Raykar et al,[47] 2015	A qualitative study exploring contextual challenges to surgical provision in 21 LMICs	*Lancet*	LMIC
Raykar et al,[67] 2016	The How Project: understanding contextual challenges to global surgical care provision in low-resource settings	*BMJ Global Health*	LMIC
Ristevski et al,[68] 2015	A qualitative study of rural women's views for the treatment of early breast cancer	*Health Expectations*	Australia
Sandelin et al,[27] 2019	Prerequisites for safe intraoperative nursing care and teamwork—operating theatre nurses' perspectives: a qualitative interview study	*Journal of Clinical Nursing*	Sweden

(continued)

First Author, y	Title	Journal	Country Represented
Scorgie et al,[37] 2010	"Cutting for love": genital incisions to enhance sexual desirability and commitment in KwaZulu-Natal, South Africa	*Reproductive Health Matters*	South Africa
Segevall et al,[69] 2019	The journey toward taking the day for granted again: the experiences of rural older people's recovery from hip fracture surgery	*Orthopaedic Nursing*	Sweden
Smith et al,[70] 2015	Australian perioperative nurses' experiences of assisting in multiorgan procurement surgery: a grounded theory study	*International Journal of Nursing Studies*	Australia
Story et al,[38] 2016	Male involvement and accommodation during obstetric emergencies in rural Ghana: a qualitative analysis	*International Perspectives on Sexual and Reproductive Health*	Ghana
Swayne & Eley,[25] 2010	Synergy and sustainability in rural procedural medicine: views from the coalface	*Australian Journal of Rural Health*	Australia
Tafida & Gilbert,[71] 2016	Exploration of indigenous knowledge systems in relation to couching in Nigeria	*African Vision and Eye Health*	Nigeria
Wade et al,[72] 2012	A qualitative study of ethical, medico-legal and clinical governance matters in Australian telehealth services	*Journal of Telemedicine and Telecare*	Australia
Wainer et al,[41] 2012	The treatment experiences of Australian women	*Reproductive Health Matters*	Australia

(continued)

First Author, y	Title	Journal	Country Represented
	with gynaecological cancers and how they can be improved: a qualitative study		
Wright et al,[73] 2011	Adoption of surgical innovations: factors influencing use of sentinel lymph node biopsy for breast cancer	*Surgical Innovation*	Canada
Youl et al,[74] 2019	What factors influence the treatment decisions of women with breast cancer? Does residential location play a role	*Rural and Remote Health*	Australia
Zhang et al,[75] 2011	Understanding barriers to cataract surgery among older persons in rural China through focus groups	*Ophthalmic Epidemiology*	China

Data from Refs.[2,7,25–41,46,47,51–75]

UNITED STATES POSTAL SERVICE®

Statement of Ownership, Management, and Circulation (All Periodicals Publications Except Requester Publications)

1. Publication Title	2. Publication Number	3. Filing Date
SURGICAL CLINICS OF NORTH AMERICA	529 – 800	9/18/2020
4. Issue Frequency	**5. Number of Issues Published Annually**	**6. Annual Subscription Price**
FEB, APR, JUN, AUG, OCT, DEC	6	$430.00

7. Complete Mailing Address of Known Office of Publication (*Not printer*) (*Street, city, county, state, and ZIP+4®*)
ELSEVIER INC.
230 Park Avenue, Suite 800
New York, NY 10169

Contact Person: Malathi Samayan
Telephone (*Include area code*): 91-44-4299-4507

8. Complete Mailing Address of Headquarters or General Business Office of Publisher (*Not printer*)
ELSEVIER INC.
230 Park Avenue, Suite 800
New York, NY 10169

9. Full Names and Complete Mailing Addresses of Publisher, Editor, and Managing Editor (*Do not leave blank*)

Publisher (*Name and complete mailing address*)
DOLORES MELONI, ELSEVIER INC.
1600 JOHN F KENNEDY BLVD. SUITE 1800
PHILADELPHIA, PA 19103-2899

Editor (*Name and complete mailing address*)
JOHN VASSALLO, ELSEVIER INC.
1600 JOHN F KENNEDY BLVD. SUITE 1800
PHILADELPHIA, PA 19103-2899

Managing Editor (*Name and complete mailing address*)
PATRICK MANLEY, ELSEVIER INC.
1600 JOHN F KENNEDY BLVD. SUITE 1800
PHILADELPHIA, PA 19103-2899

10. Owner (*Do not leave blank. If the publication is owned by a corporation, give the name and address of the corporation immediately followed by the names and addresses of all stockholders owning or holding 1 percent or more of the total amount of stock. If not owned by a corporation, give the names and addresses of the individual owners. If owned by a partnership or other unincorporated firm, give its name and address as well as those of each individual owner. If the publication is published by a nonprofit organization, give its name and address.*)

Full Name	Complete Mailing Address
WHOLLY OWNED SUBSIDIARY OF REED/ELSEVIER, US HOLDINGS	1600 JOHN F KENNEDY BLVD. SUITE 1800 PHILADELPHIA, PA 19103-2899

11. Known Bondholders, Mortgagees, and Other Security Holders Owning or Holding 1 Percent or More of Total Amount of Bonds, Mortgages, or Other Securities. If none, check box → ☐ None

Full Name	Complete Mailing Address
N/A	

12. Tax Status (*For completion by nonprofit organizations authorized to mail at nonprofit rates*) (*Check one*)
The purpose, function, and nonprofit status of this organization and the exempt status for federal income tax purposes:
☒ Has Not Changed During Preceding 12 Months
☐ Has Changed During Preceding 12 Months (*Publisher must submit explanation of change with this statement*)

13. Publication Title	14. Issue Date for Circulation Data Below
SURGICAL CLINICS OF NORTH AMERICA	JUNE 2020

15. Extent and Nature of Circulation			Average No. Copies Each Issue During Preceding 12 Months	No. Copies of Single Issue Published Nearest to Filing Date
a. Total Number of Copies (*Net press run*)			399	332
b. Paid Circulation (*By Mail and Outside the Mail*)	(1)	Mailed Outside-County Paid Subscriptions Stated on PS Form 3541 (Include paid distribution above nominal rate, advertiser's proof copies, and exchange copies)	186	156
	(2)	Mailed In-County Paid Subscriptions Stated on PS Form 3541 (*Include paid distribution above nominal rate, advertiser's proof copies, and exchange copies*)	0	0
	(3)	Paid Distribution Outside the Mails Including Sales Through Dealers and Carriers, Street Vendors, Counter Sales, and Other Paid Distribution Outside USPS®	169	136
	(4)	Paid Distribution by Other Classes of Mail Through the USPS (e.g., First-Class Mail®)	0	0
c. Total Paid Distribution [*Sum of 15b (1), (2), (3), and (4)*] ▶			355	292
d. Free or Nominal Rate Distribution (*By Mail and Outside the Mail*)	(1)	Free or Nominal Rate Outside-County Copies included on PS Form 3541	24	19
	(2)	Free or Nominal Rate In-County Copies Included on PS Form 3541	0	0
	(3)	Free or Nominal Rate Copies Mailed at Other Classes Through the USPS (e.g., First-Class Mail)	0	0
	(4)	Free or Nominal Rate Distribution Outside the Mail (*Carriers or other means*)	0	0
e. Total Free or Nominal Rate Distribution (*Sum of 15d (1), (2), (3) and (4)*)			24	19
f. Total Distribution (*Sum of 15c and 15e*) ▶			379	311
g. Copies not Distributed (*See Instructions to Publishers #4 (page #3)*) ▶			20	21
h. Total (*Sum of 15f and g*)			399	332
i. Percent Paid (*15c divided by 15f times 100*) ▶			93.66%	93.89%

* If you are claiming electronic copies, go to line 16 on page 3. If you are not claiming electronic copies, skip to line 17 on page 3.

16. Electronic Copy Circulation	Average No. Copies Each Issue During Preceding 12 Months	No. Copies of Single Issue Published Nearest to Filing Date
a. Paid Electronic Copies ▶		
b. Total Paid Print Copies (Line 15c) + Paid Electronic Copies (Line 16a) ▶		
c. Total Print Distribution (Line 15f) + Paid Electronic Copies (Line 16a) ▶		
d. Percent Paid (Both Print & Electronic Copies) (16b divided by 16c × 100) ▶		

☒ **I certify that 50% of all my distributed copies (electronic and print) are paid above a nominal price.**

17. Publication of Statement of Ownership

☒ If the publication is a general publication, publication of this statement is required. Will be printed in the OCTOBER 2020 issue of this publication. ☐ Publication not required.

18. Signature and Title of Editor, Publisher, Business Manager, or Owner

Malathi Samayan - Distribution Controller — *Malathi Samayan* — Date: 9/18/2020

I certify that all information furnished on this form is true and complete. I understand that anyone who furnishes false or misleading information on this form or who omits material or information requested on the form may be subject to criminal sanctions (including fines and imprisonment) and/or civil sanctions (including civil penalties).

Printed and bound by CPI Group (UK) Ltd, Croydon, CR0 4YY
03/10/2024
01040484-0016